Contents

Trace the lines
Trace the shapes
Trace the letters
Trace the numbers

Trace and match
Connect the dots
Symmetry drawing
Shadow matching
Item hunt
Coloring pages
Continue the pattern
Eye-hand coordination
Spot differences
Mazes
Word scramble
Telling time
Sudoku
Find two same pictures

Trace the lines

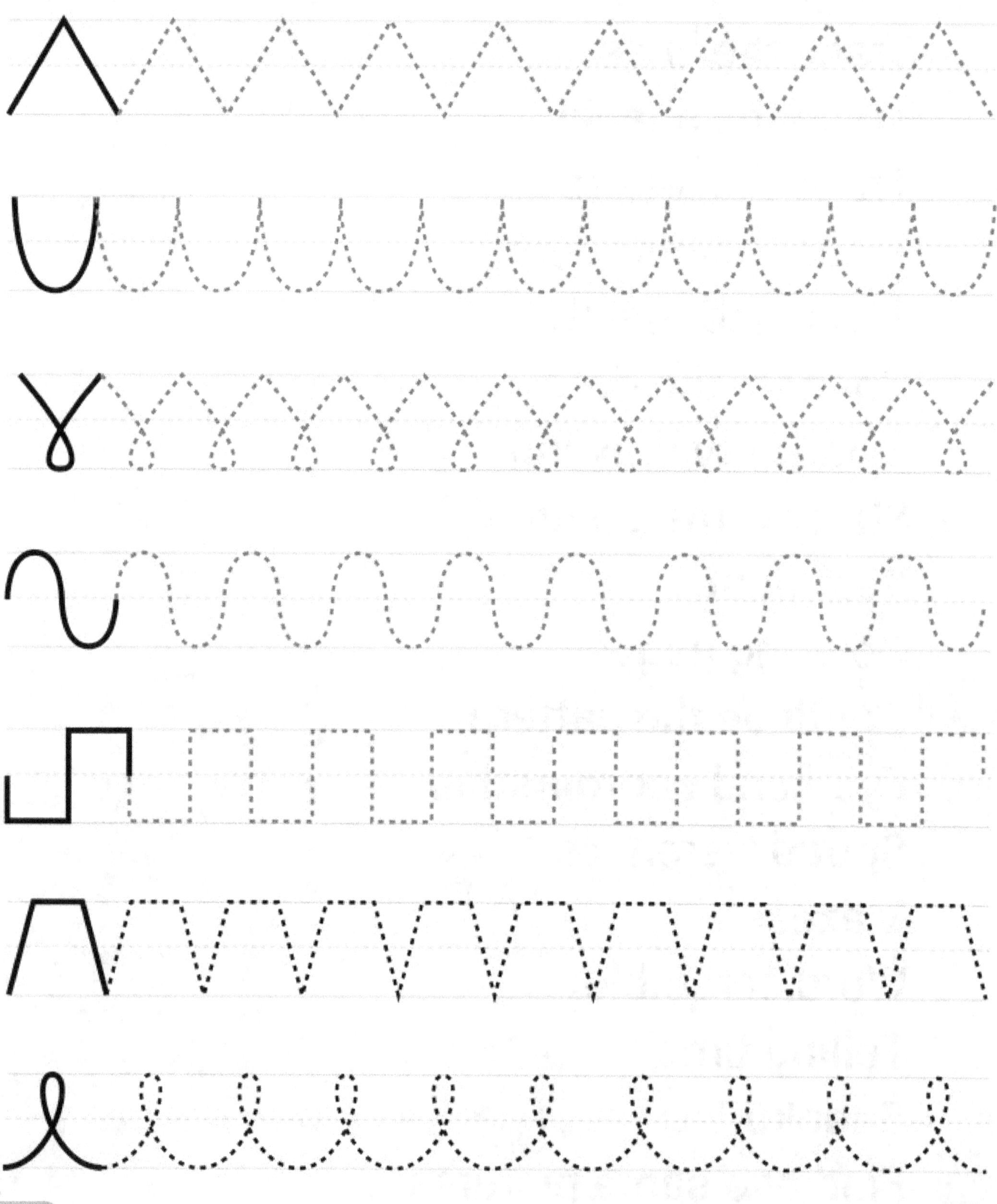

Trace the lines

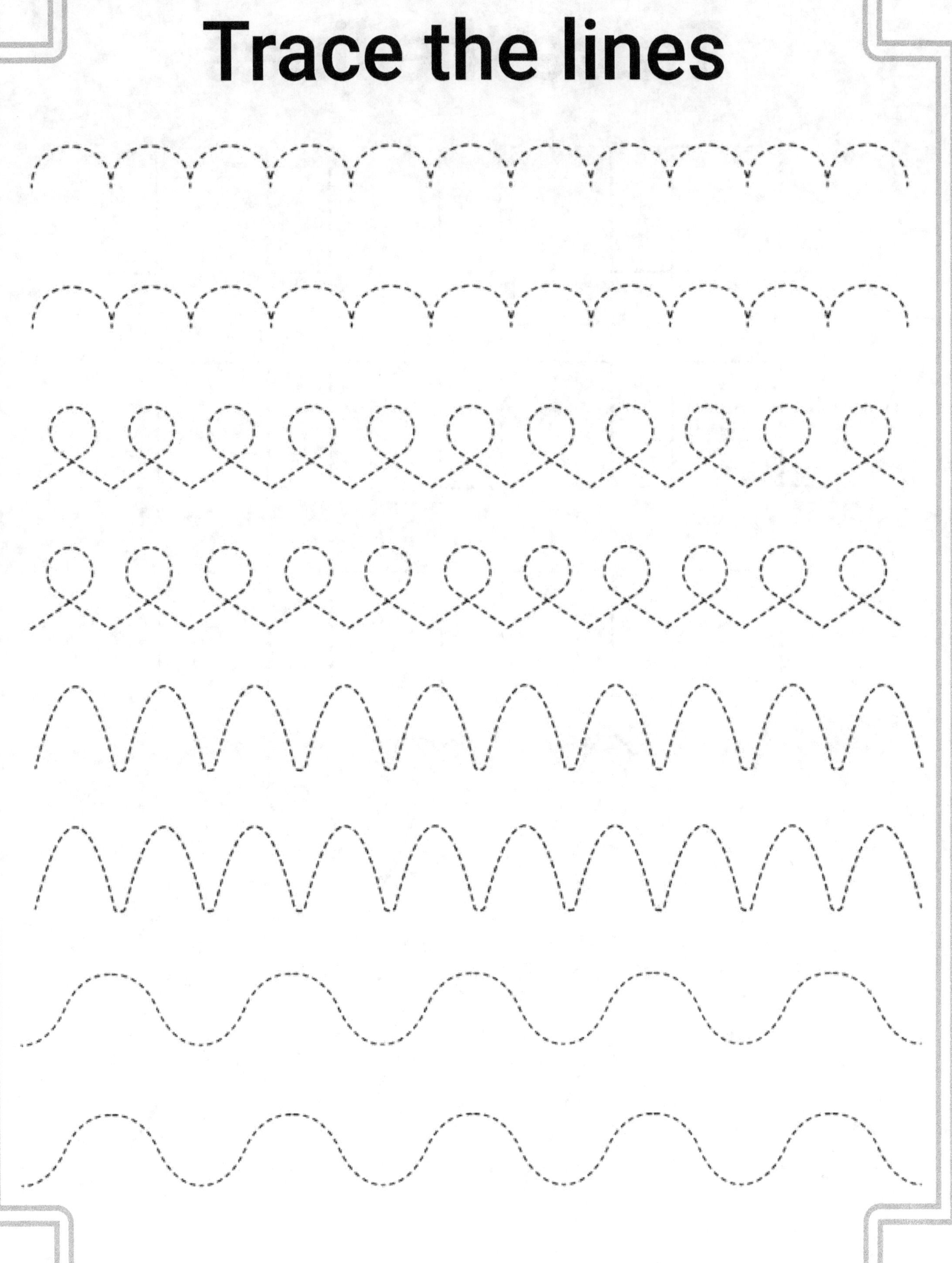

Trace the lines

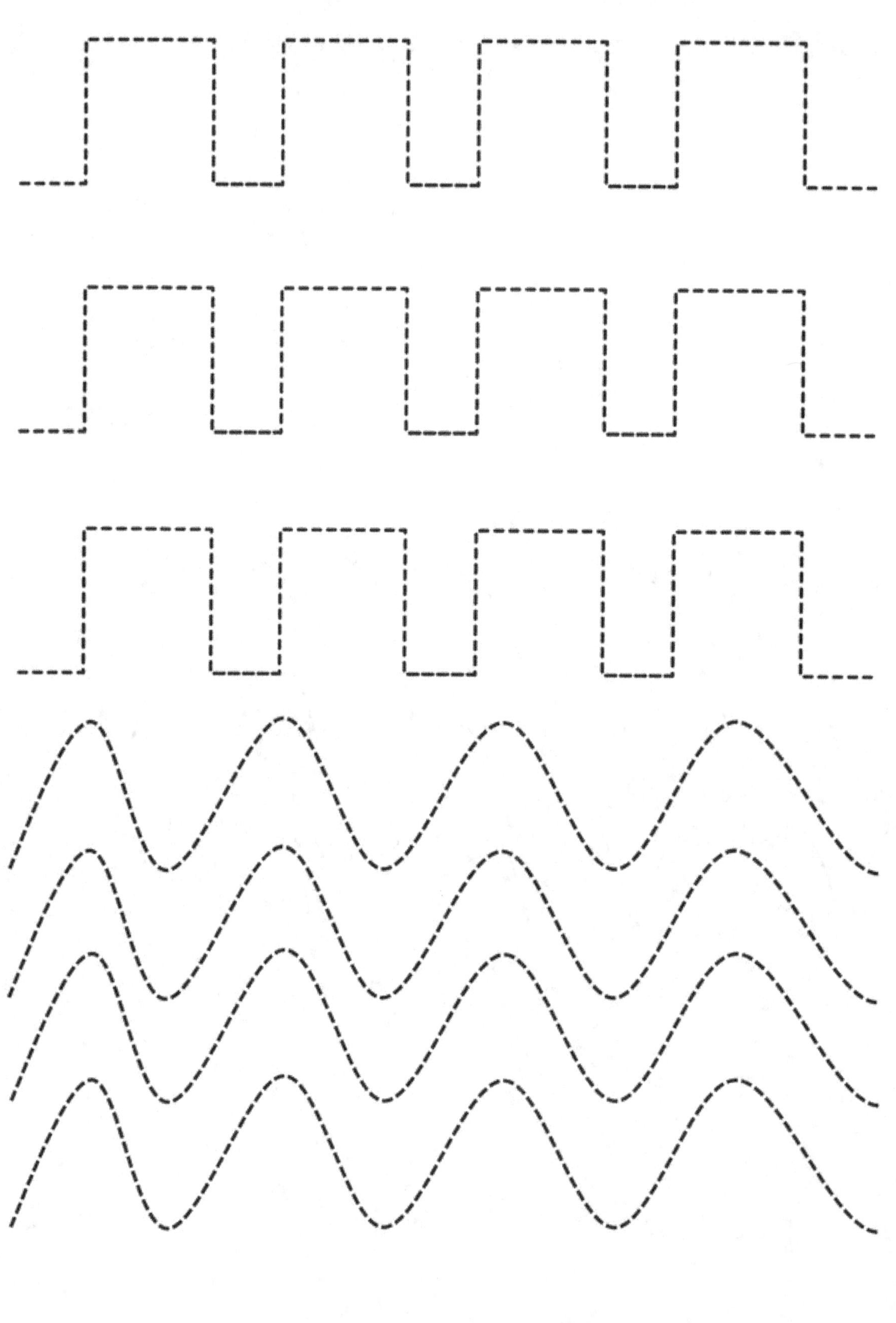

Trace the shapes

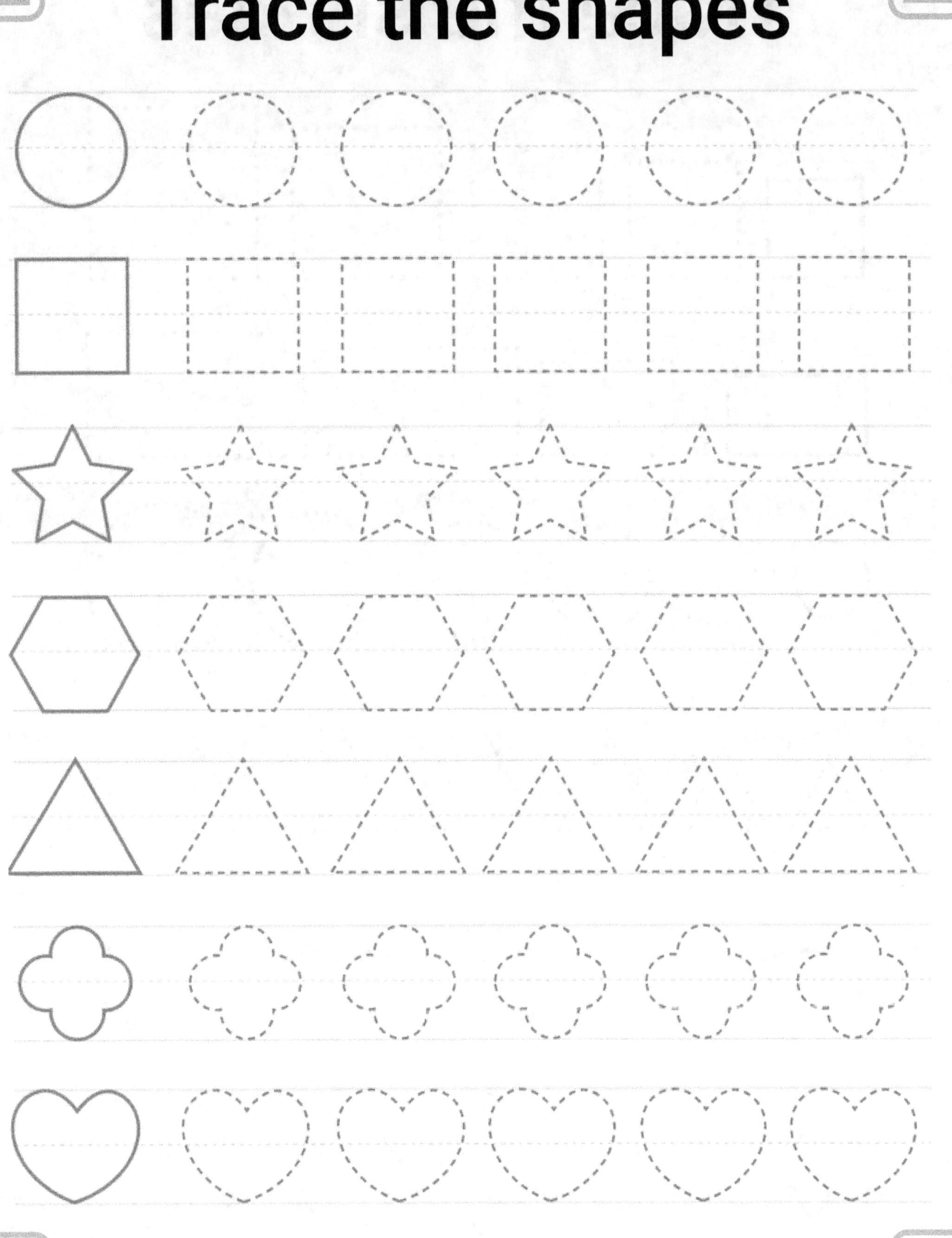

Trace the shapes

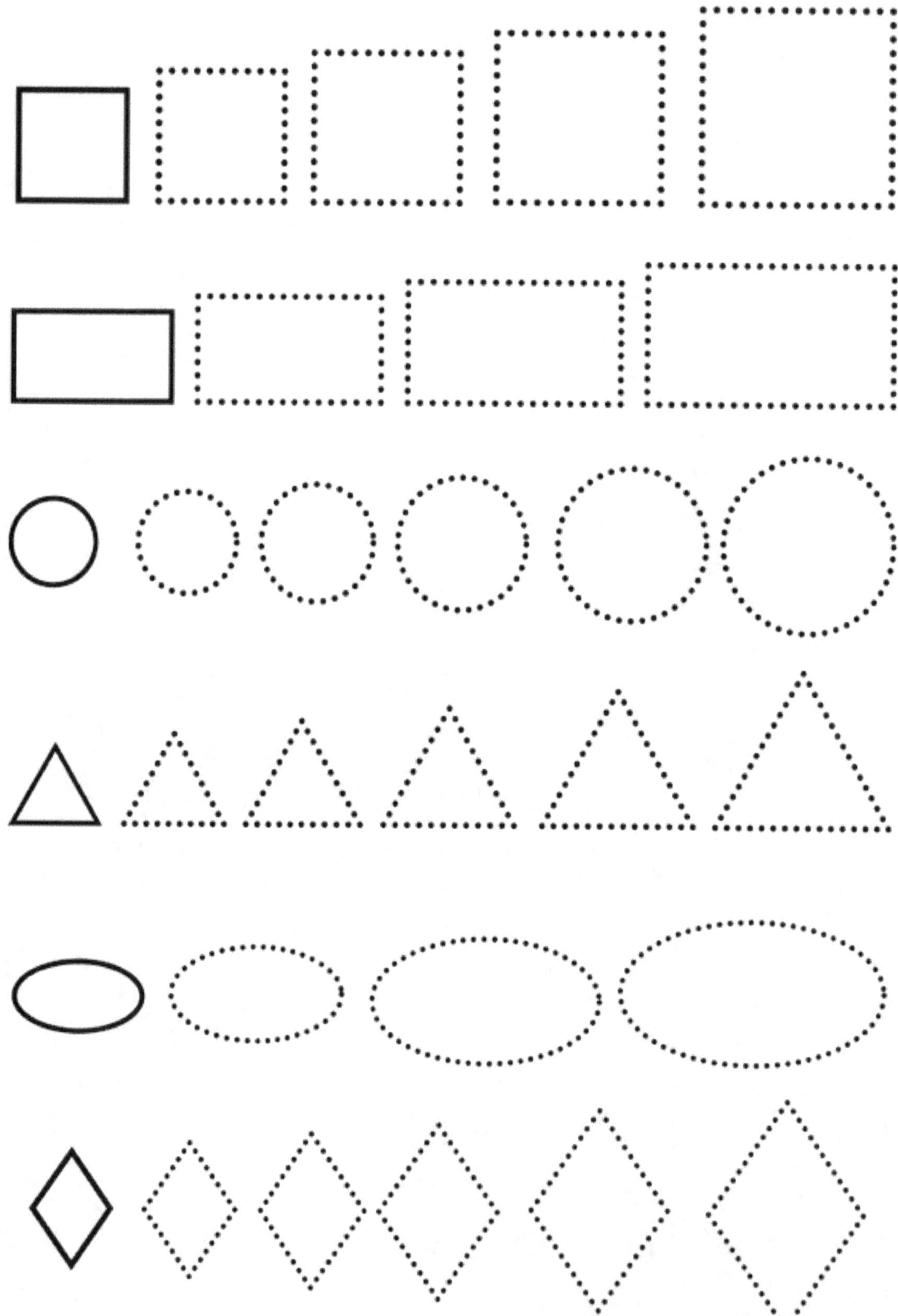

Trace the shapes

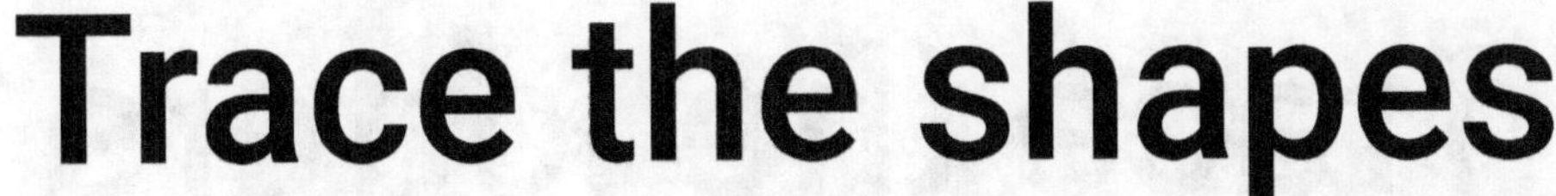

CIRCLE   SQUARE 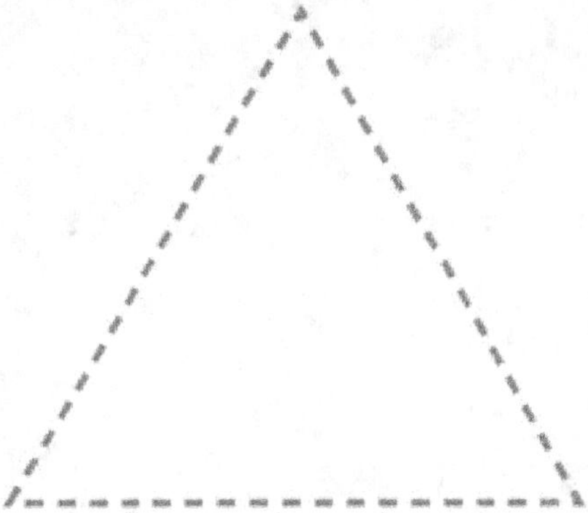   TRIANGLE

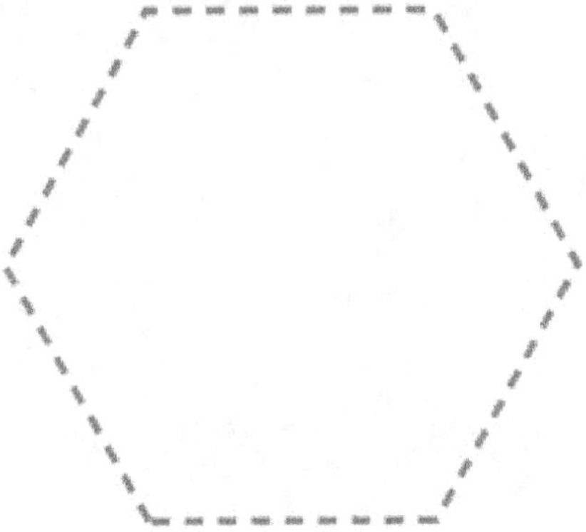

HEXAGON   RECTANGLE 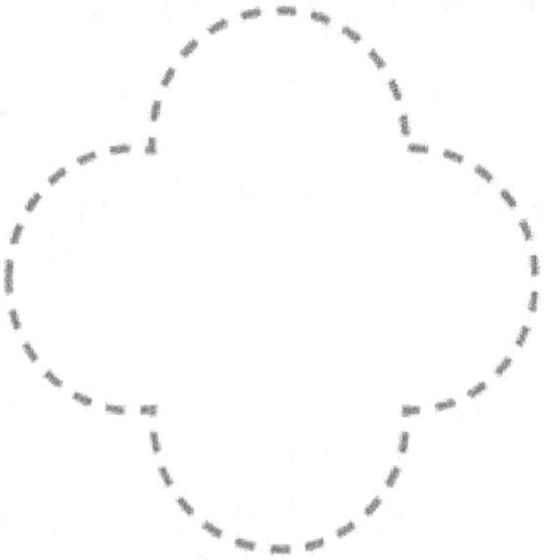   QUATREFOIL

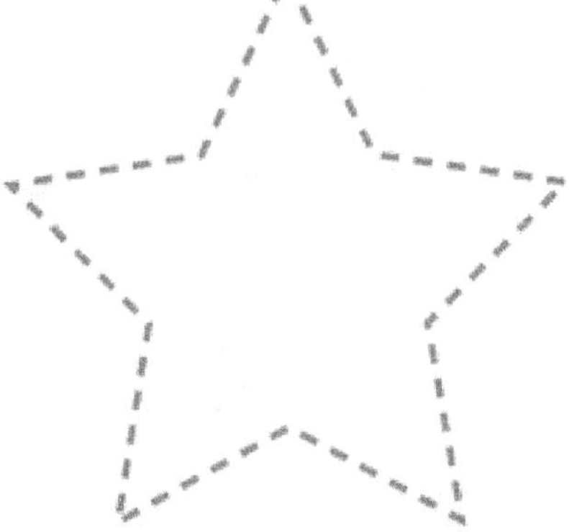

STAR 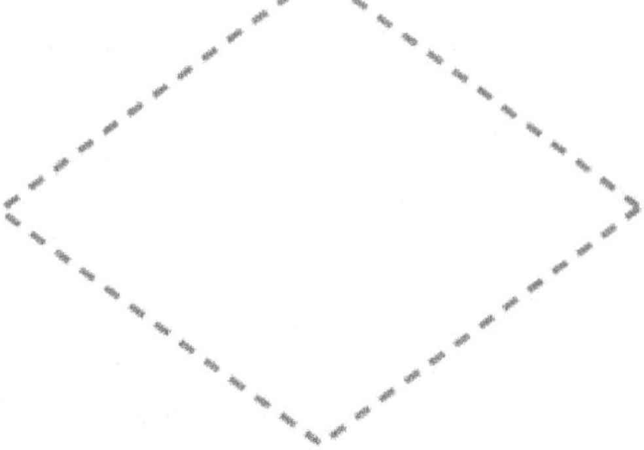   DIAMOND 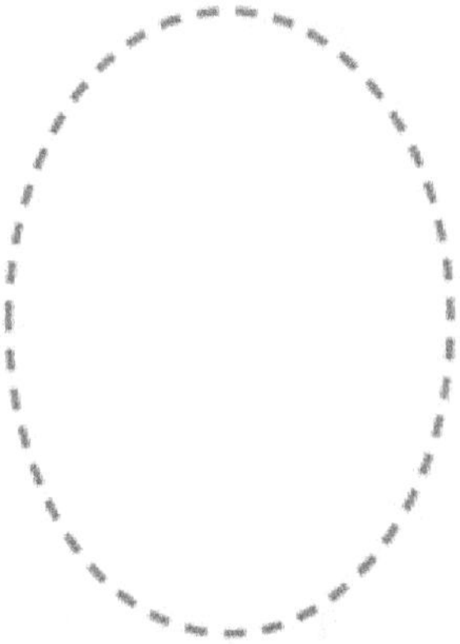   OVAL

Trace the letters

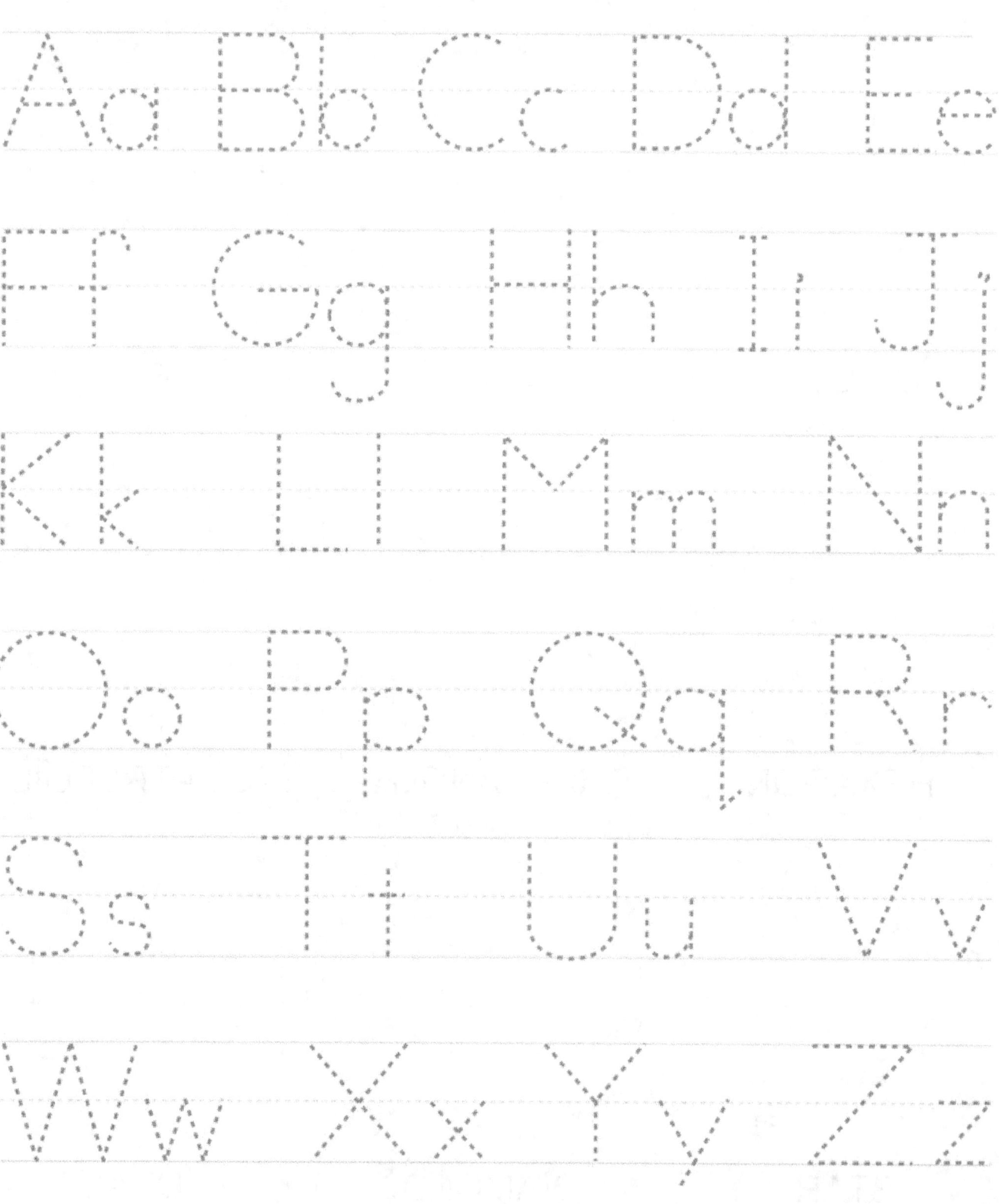

Trace the letters

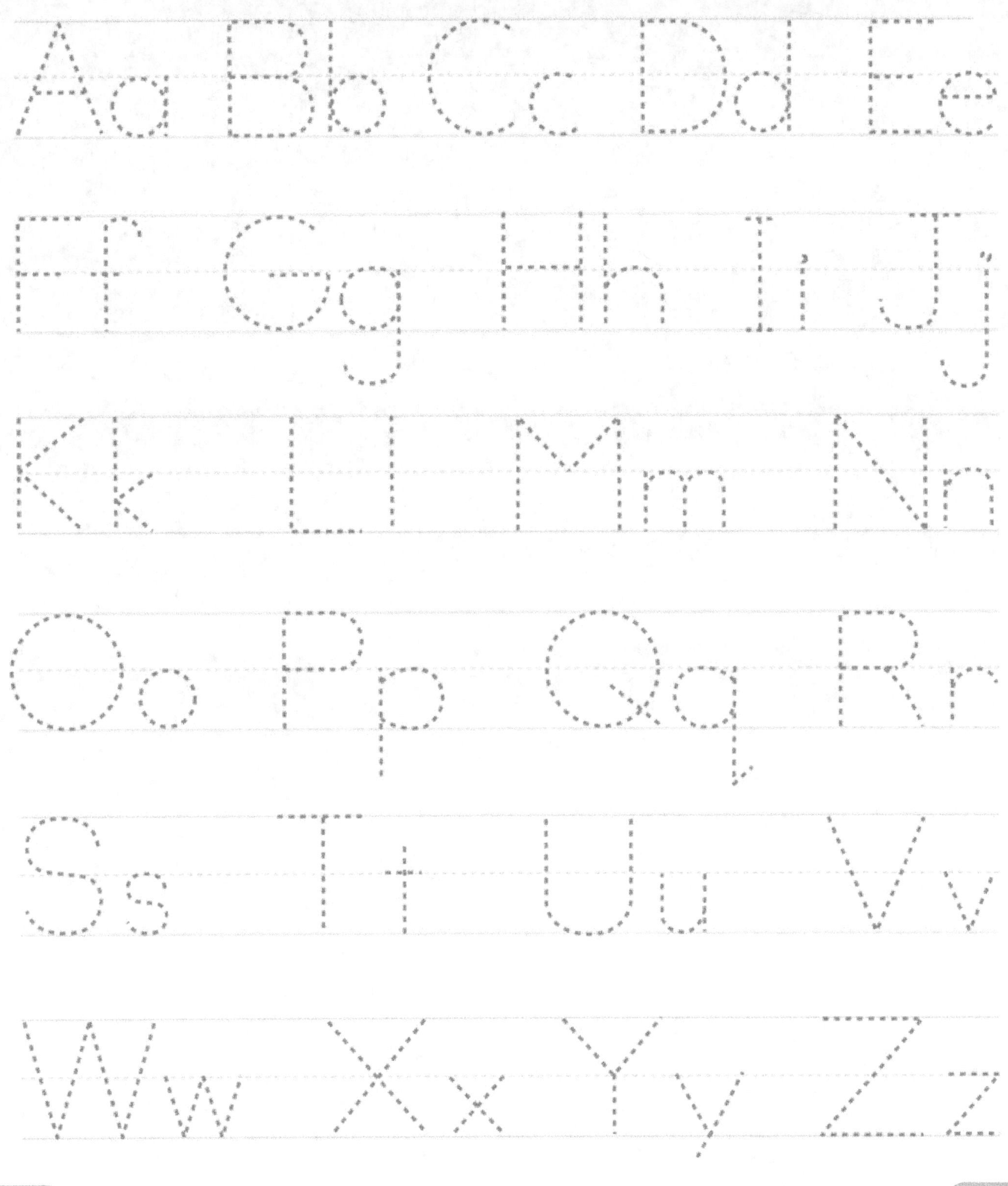

Trace the letters

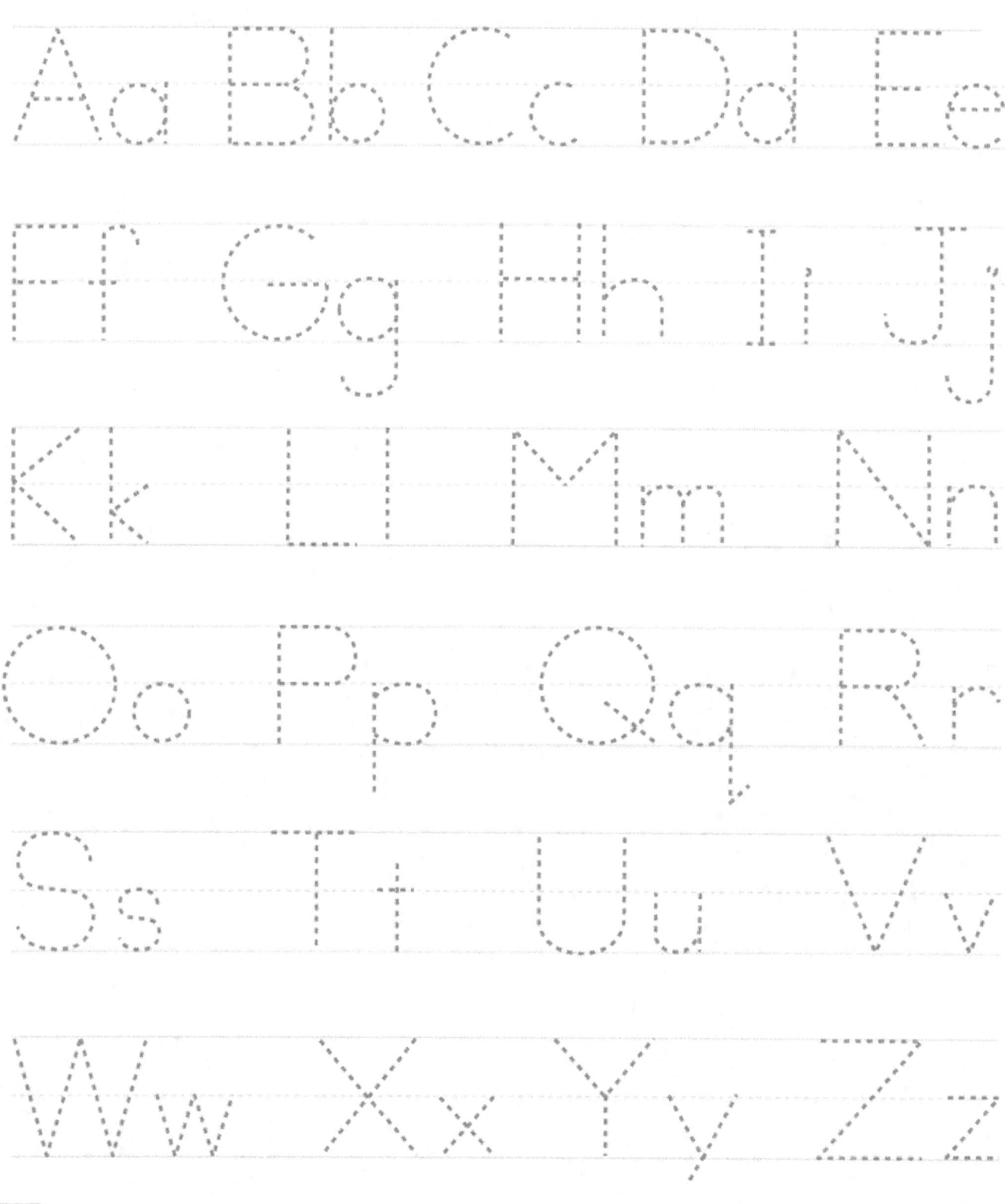

Trace the numbers

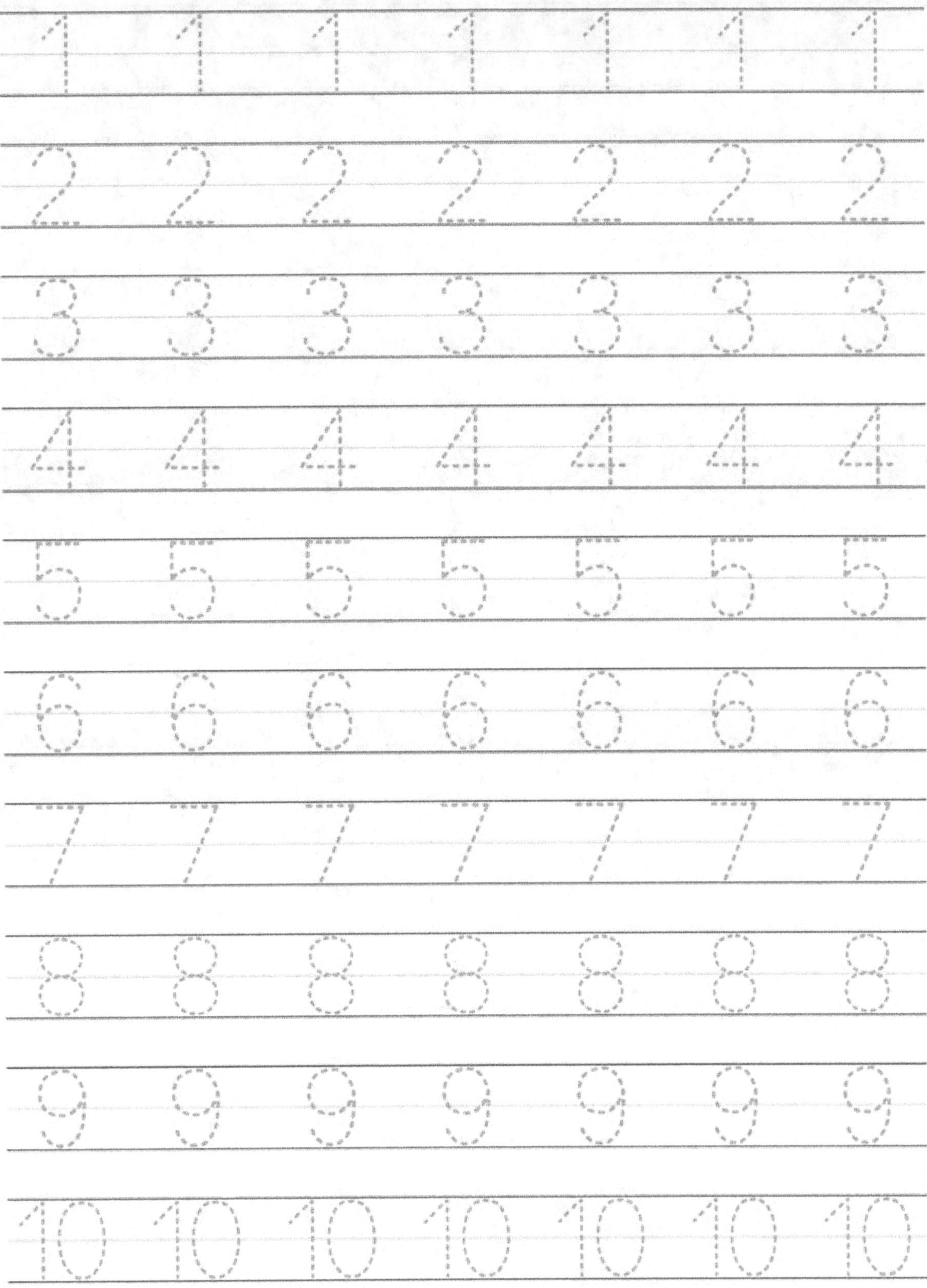

Trace the numbers

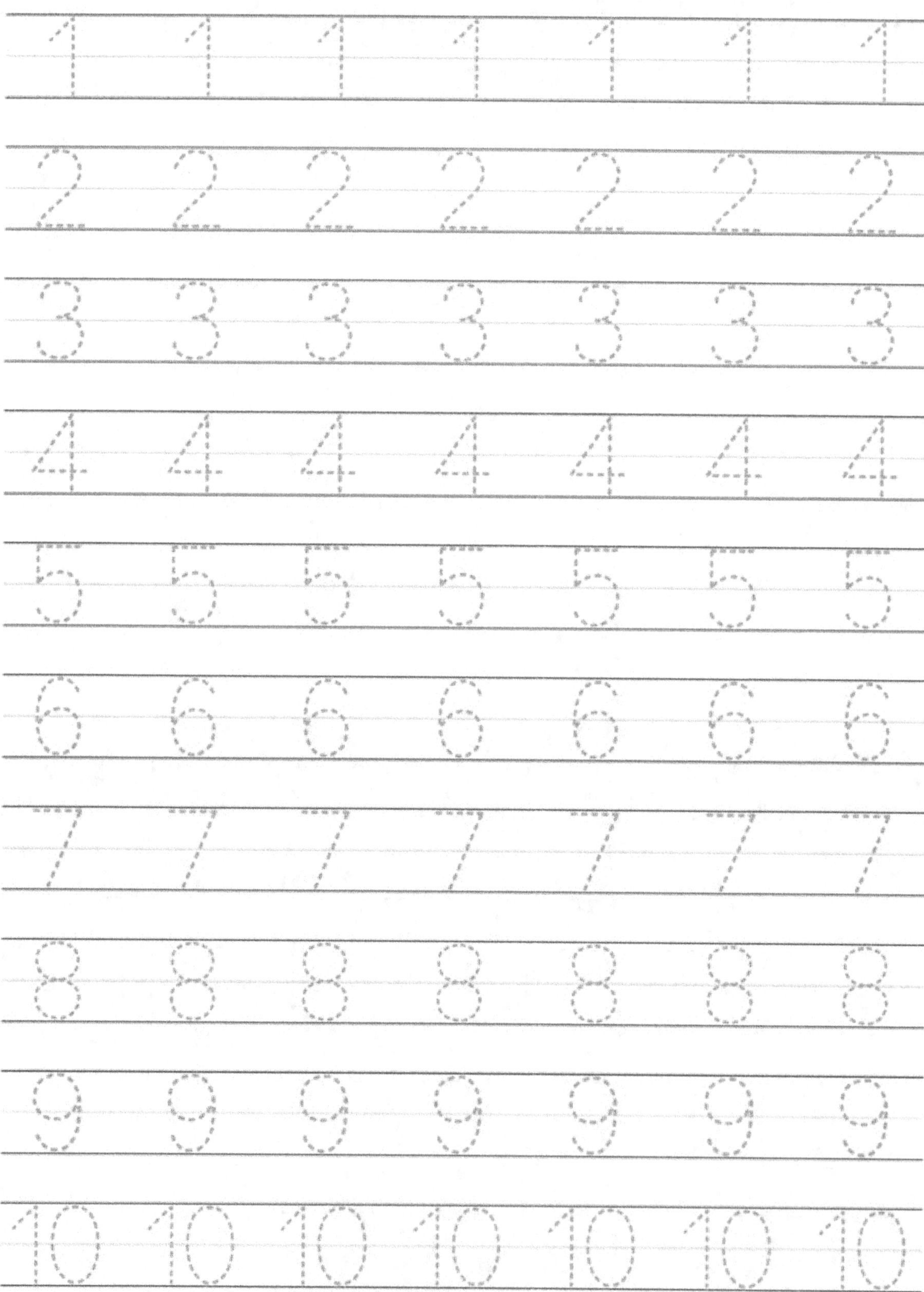

Trace the numbers

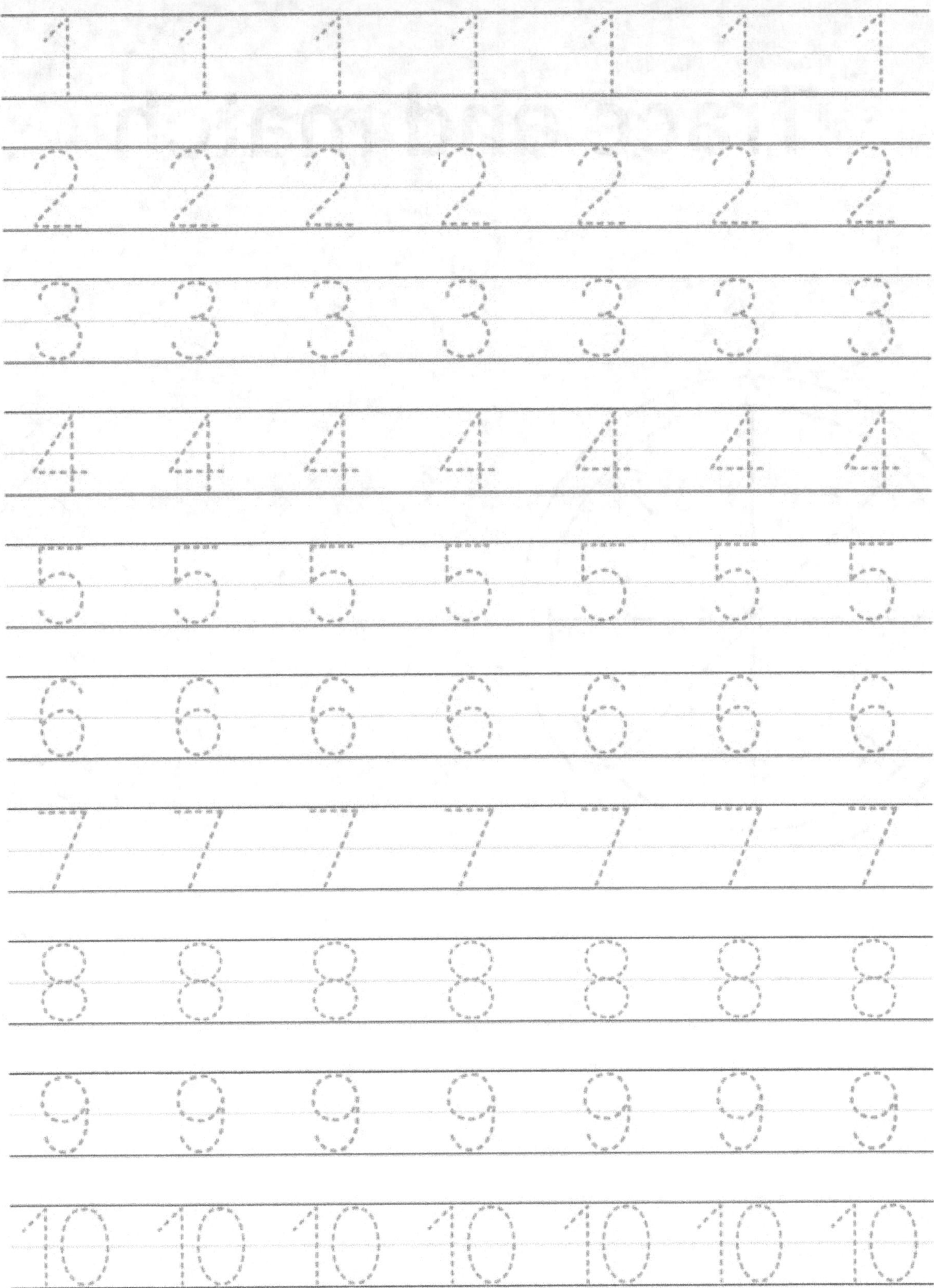

Trace and match

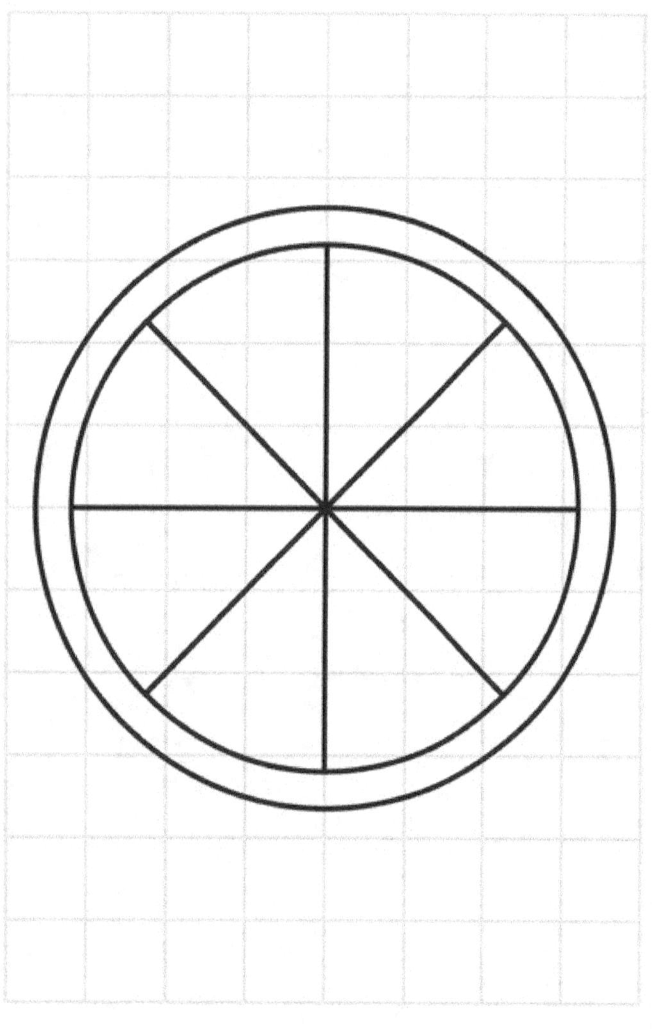 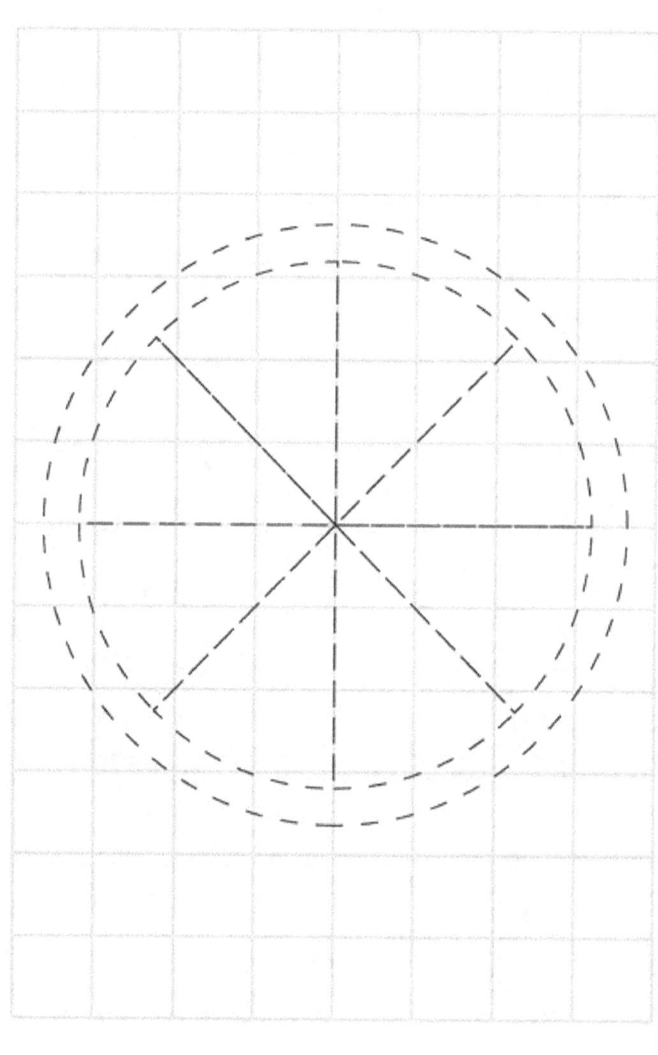

Trace and match

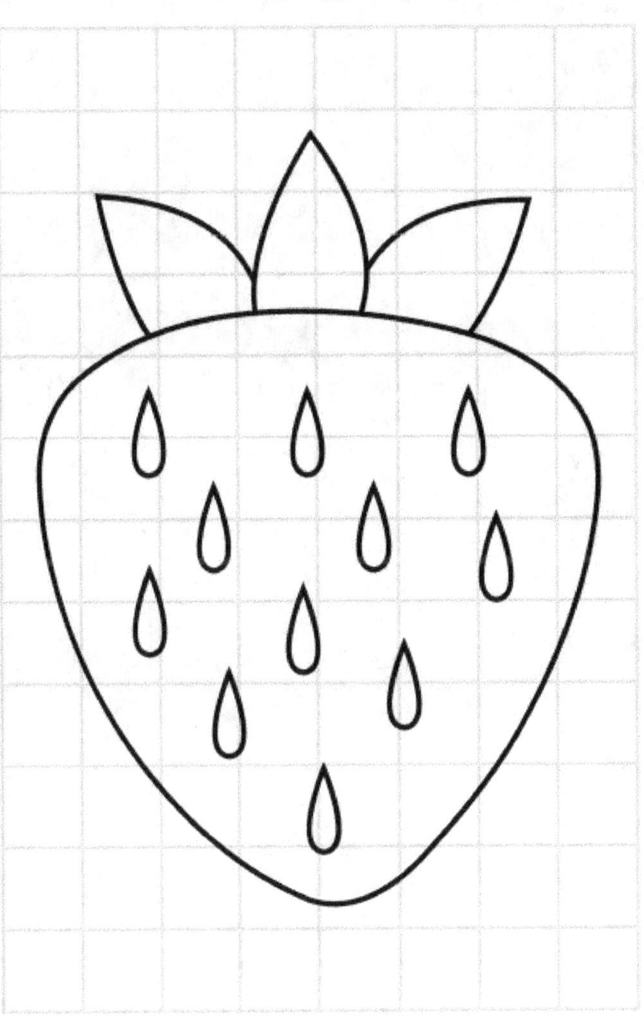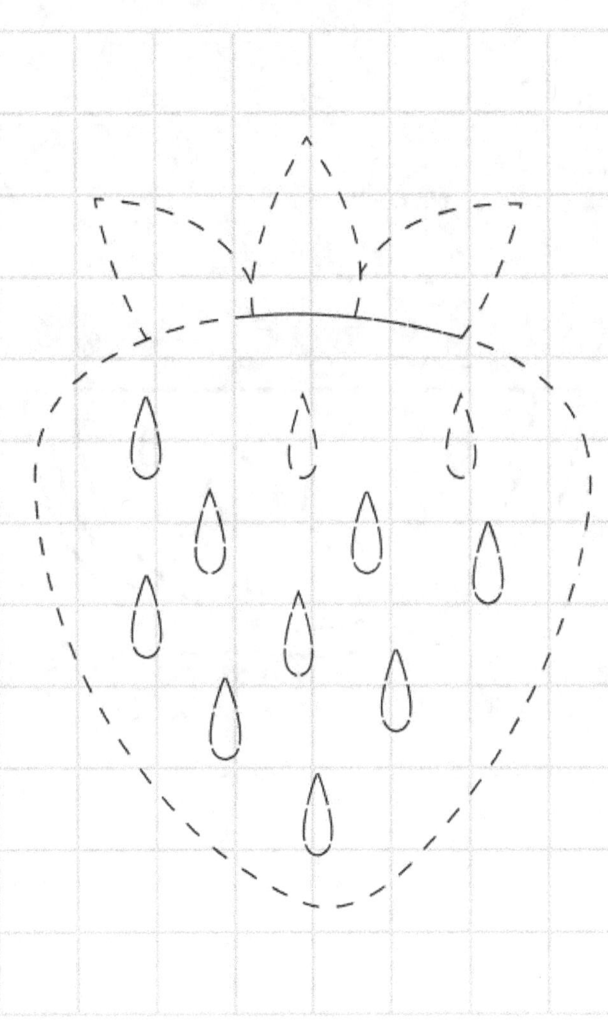

Trace and match

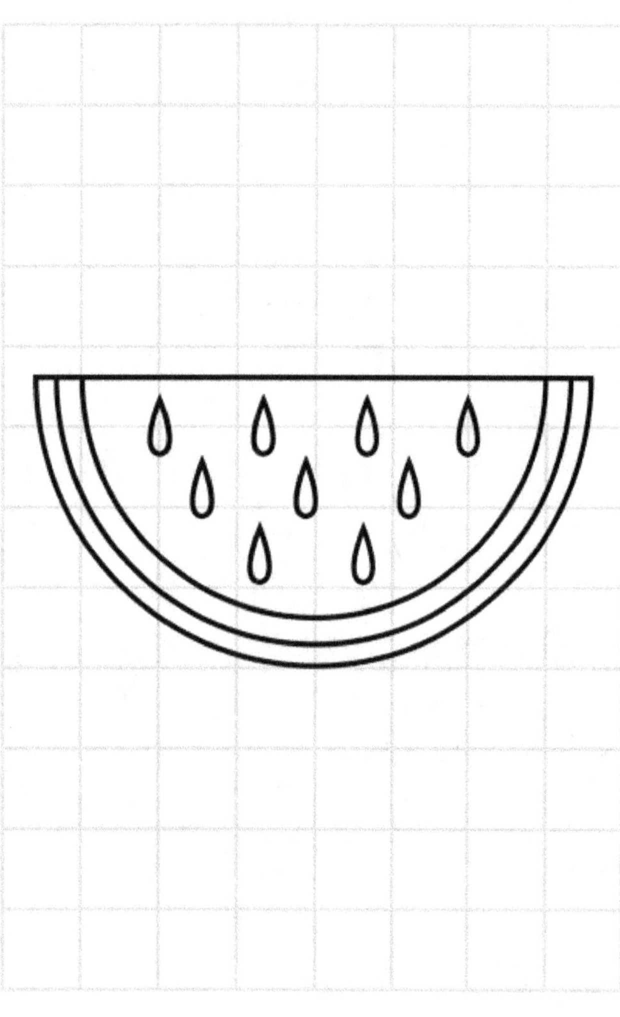 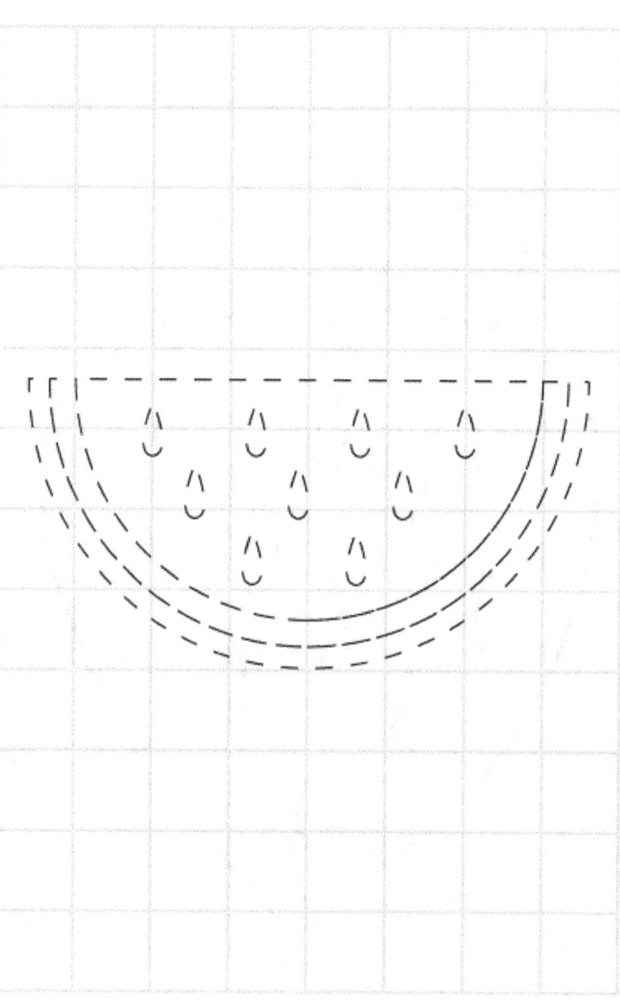

Connect the dots

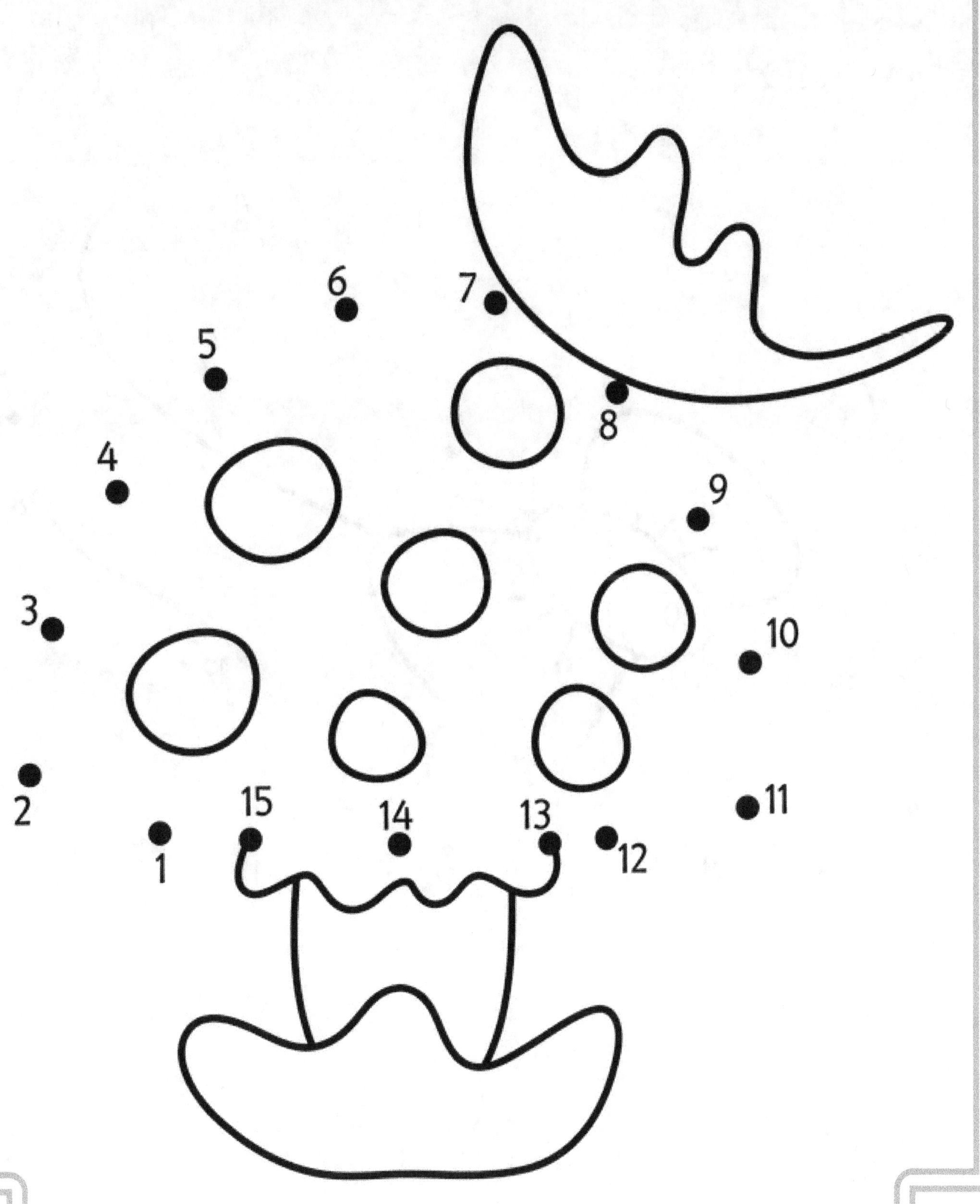

Connect the dots

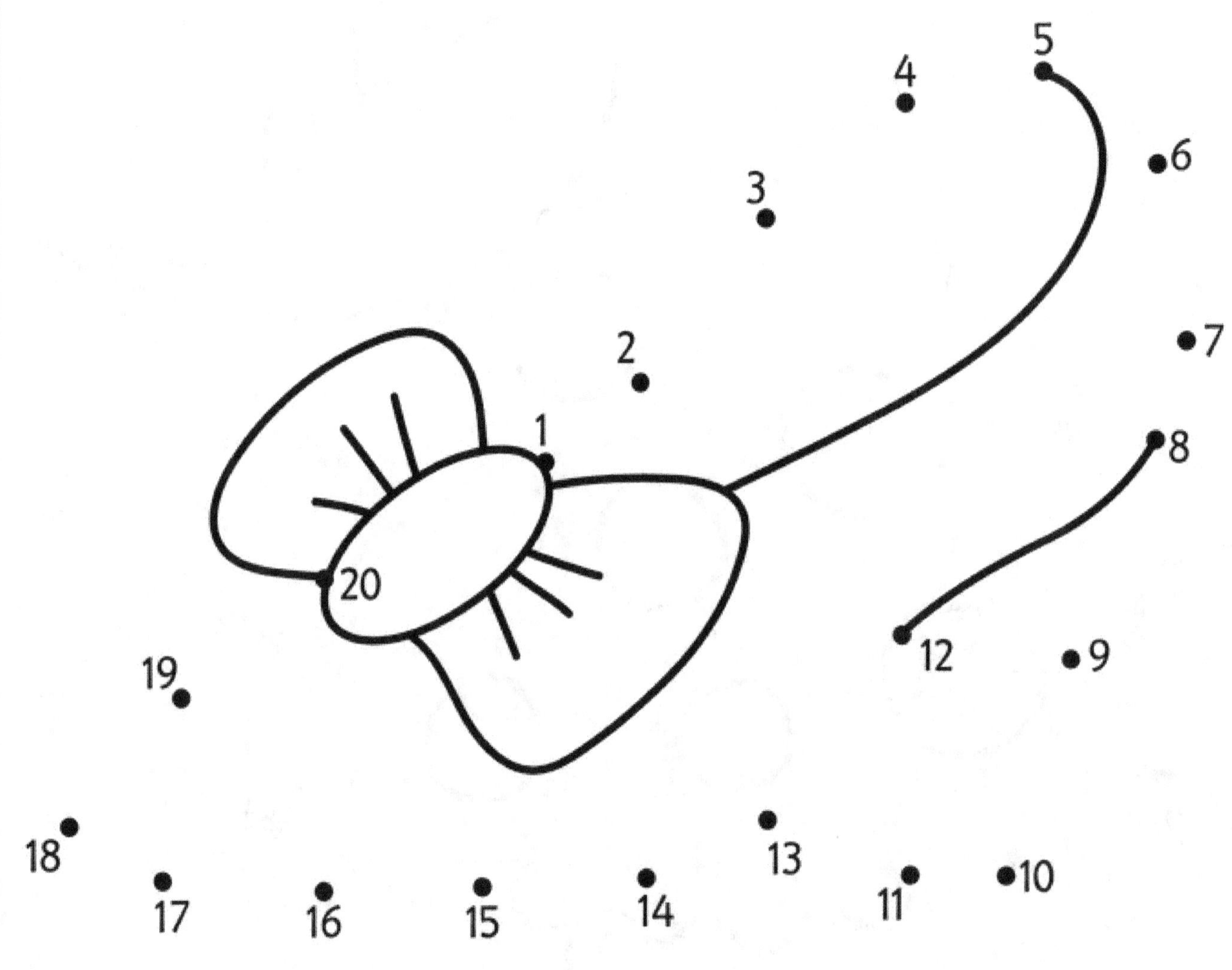

Connect the dots

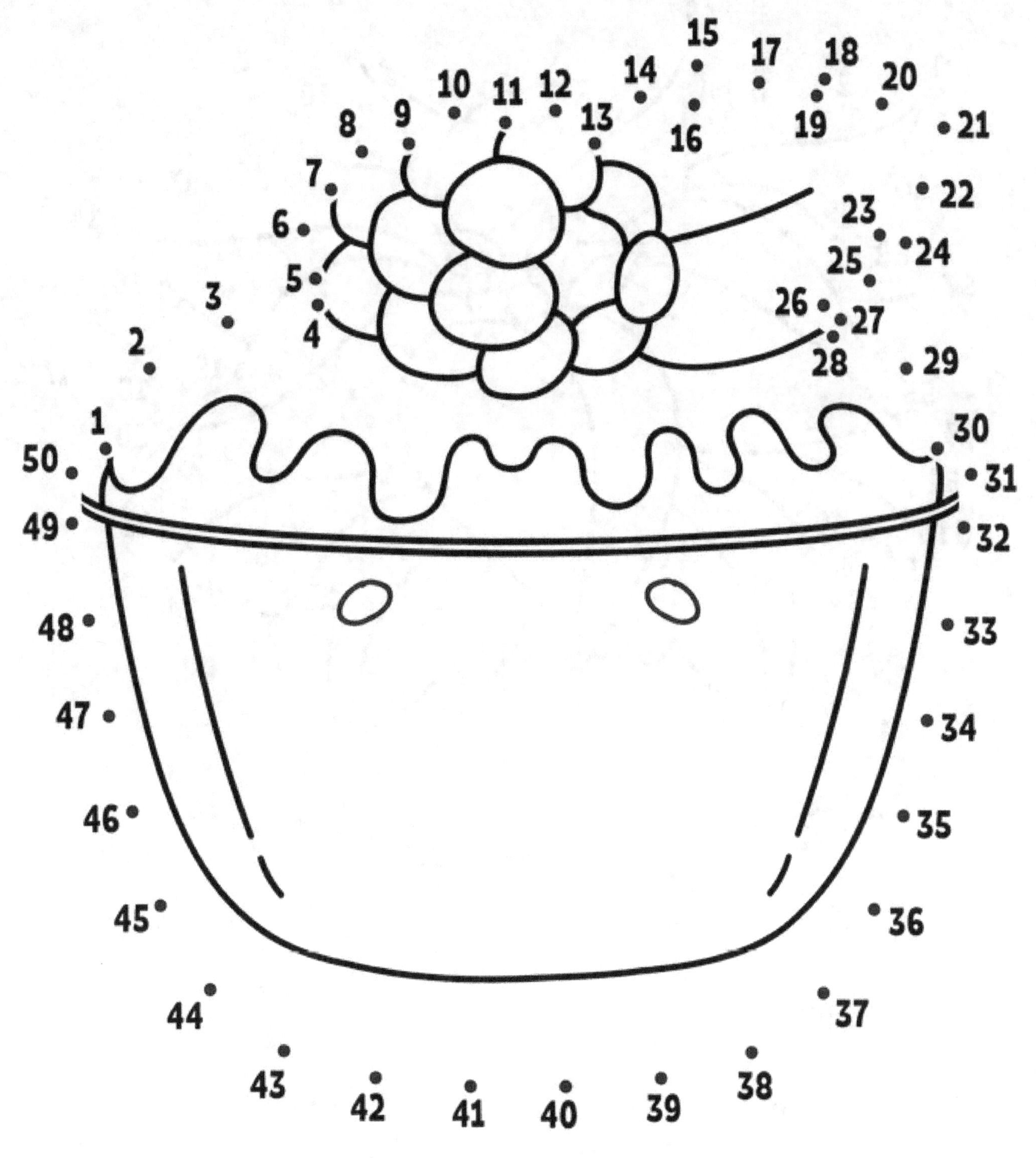

Connect the dots

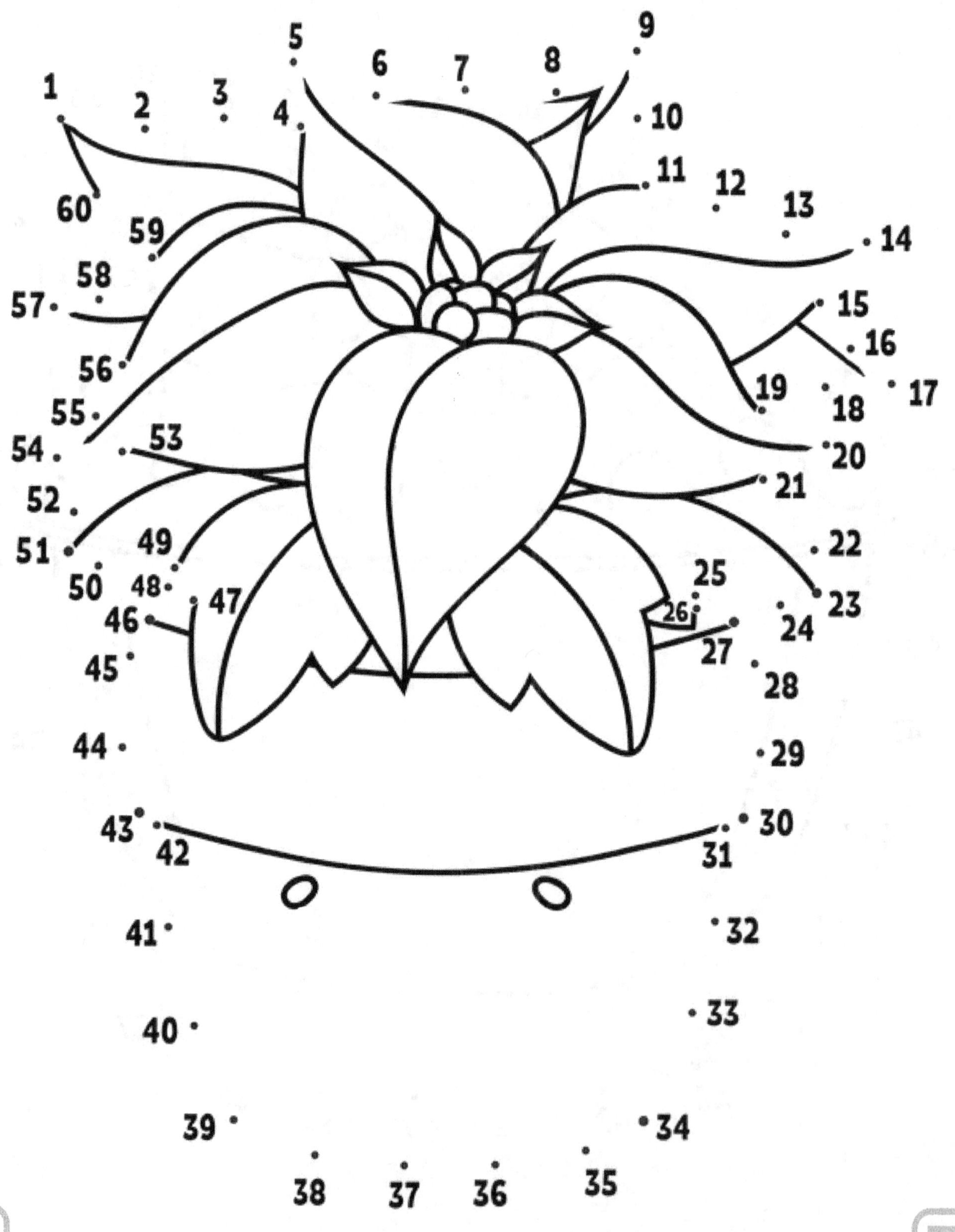

Symmetry drawing

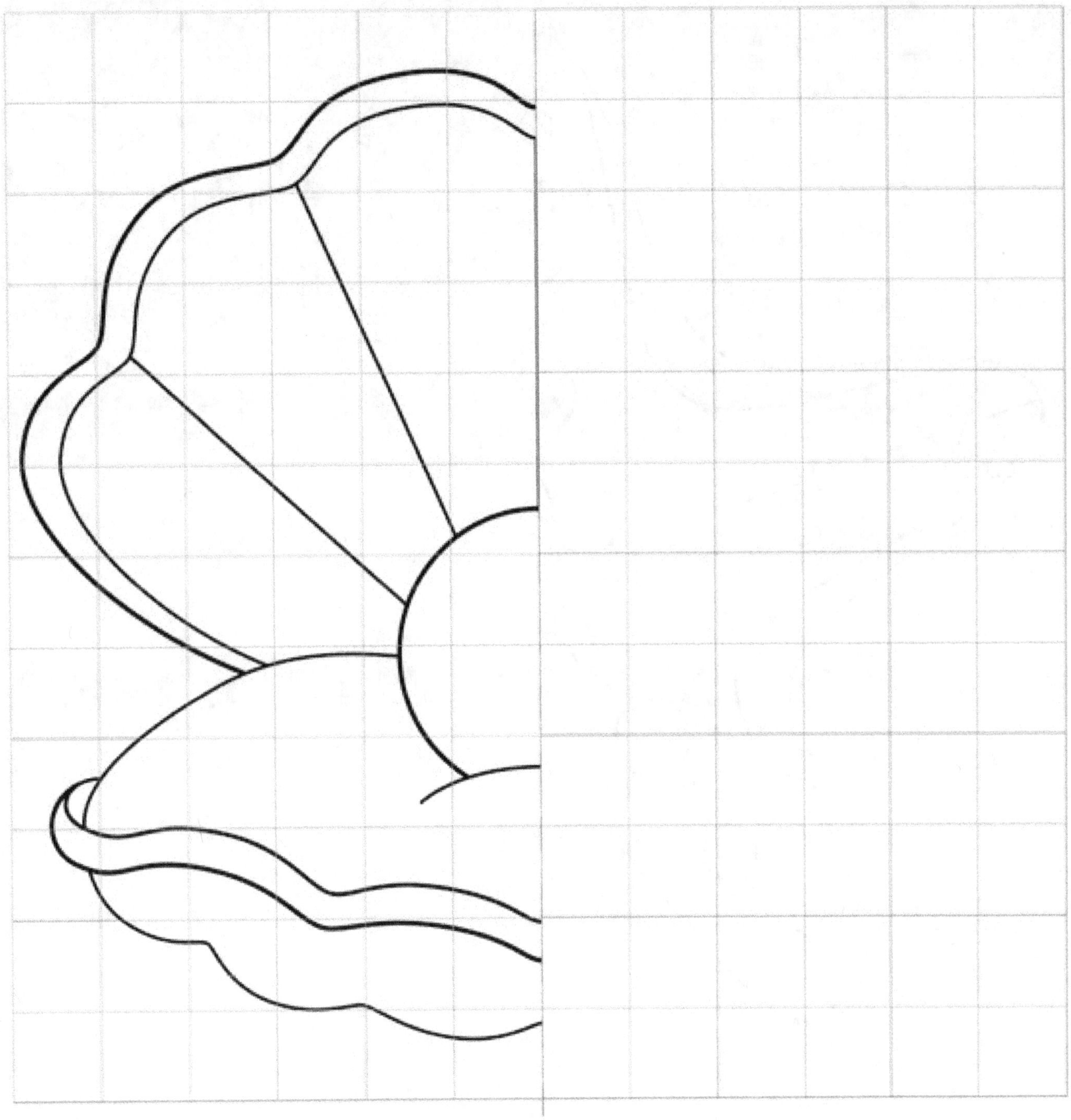

Symmetry drawing

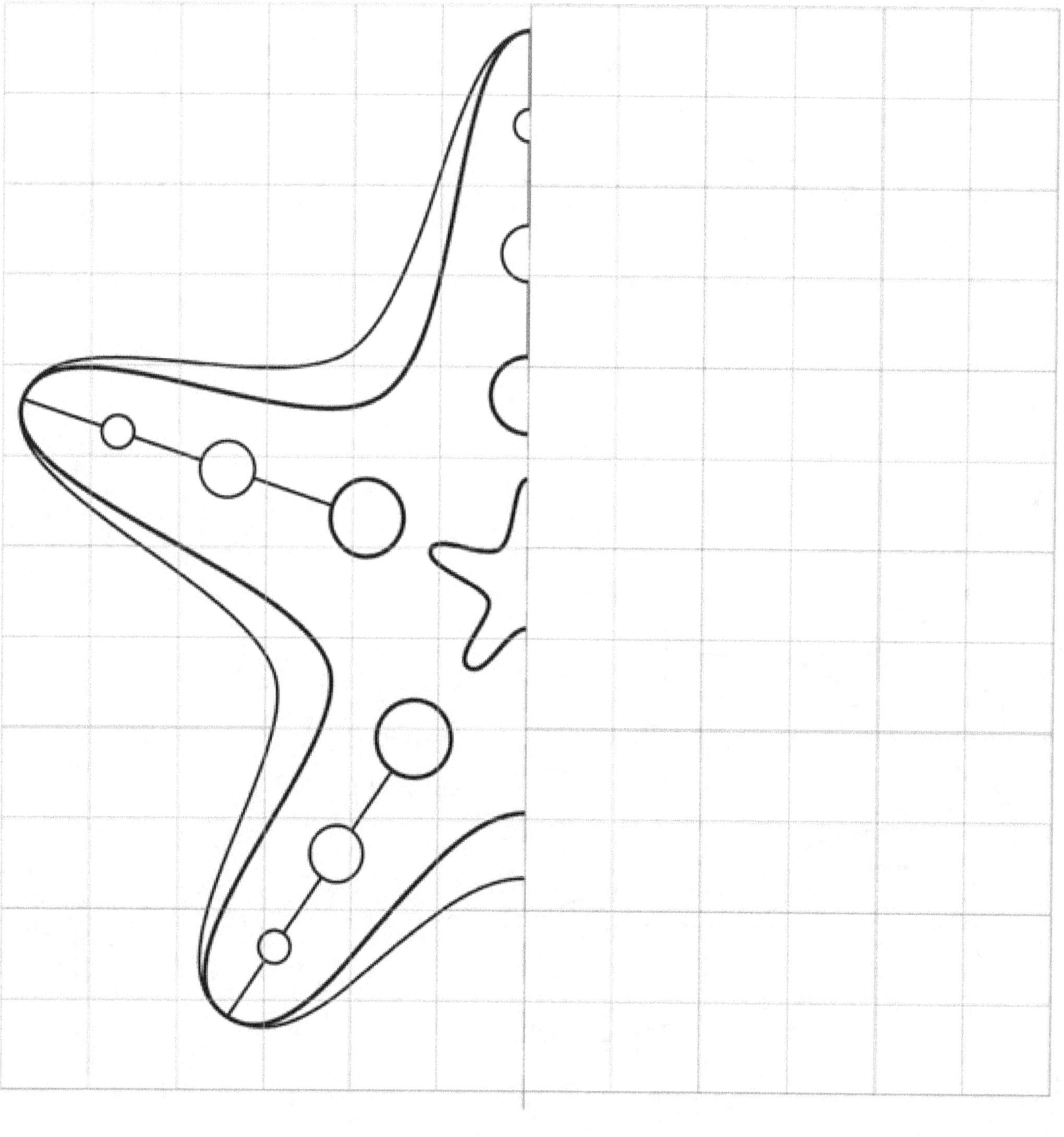

Symmetry drawing

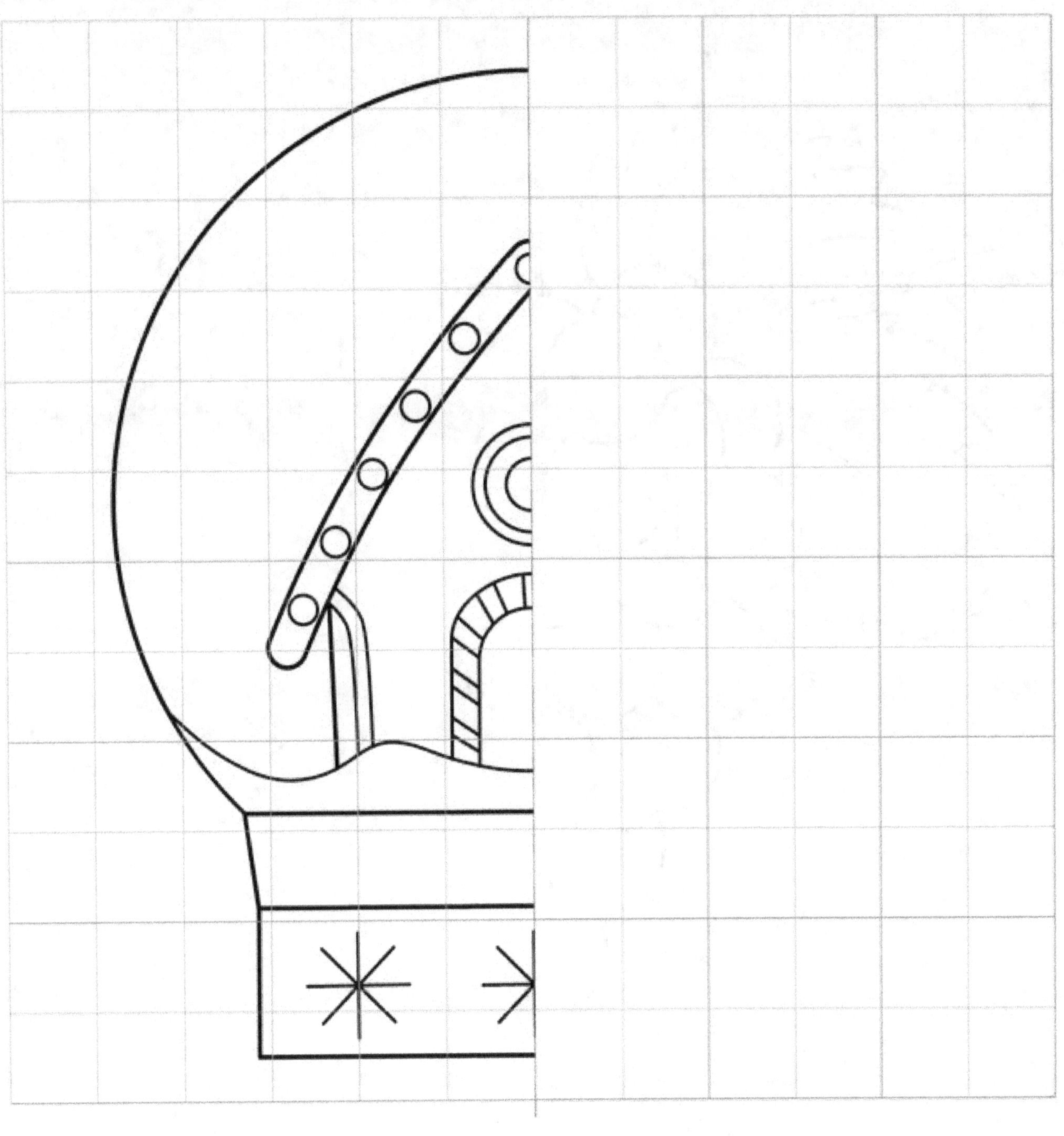

Symmetry drawing

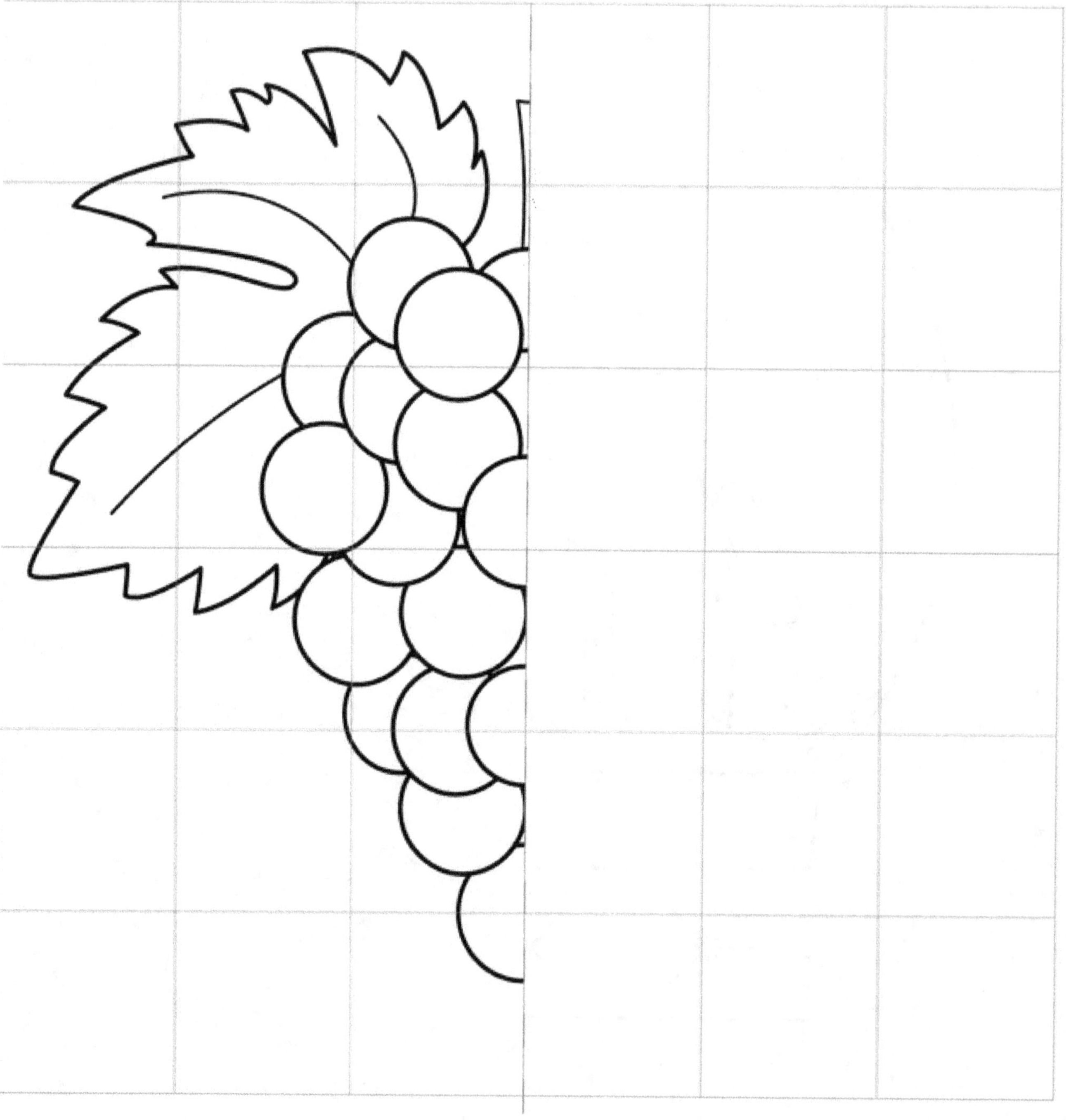

Shadow matching

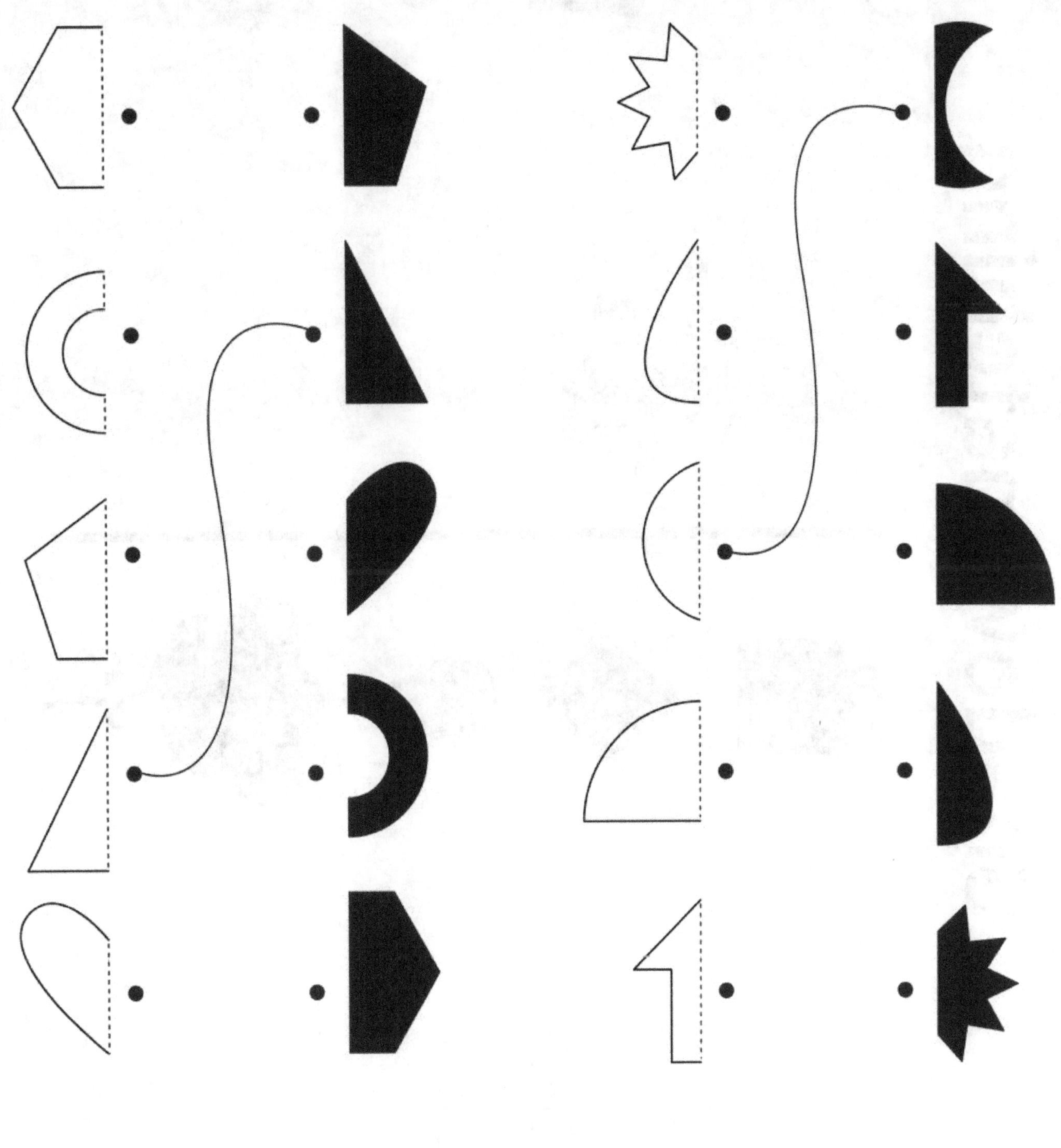

Shadow matching

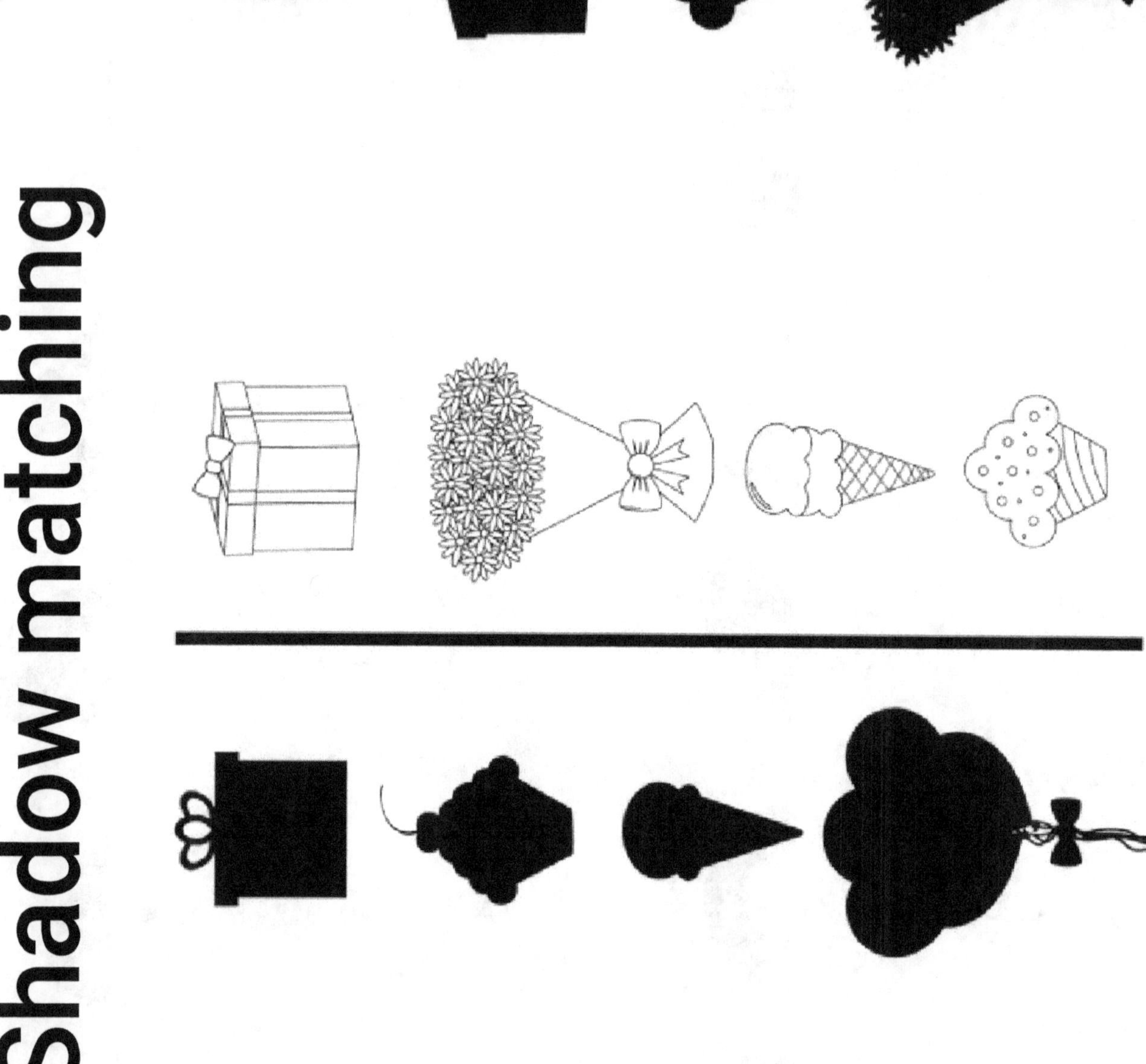

Shadow matching

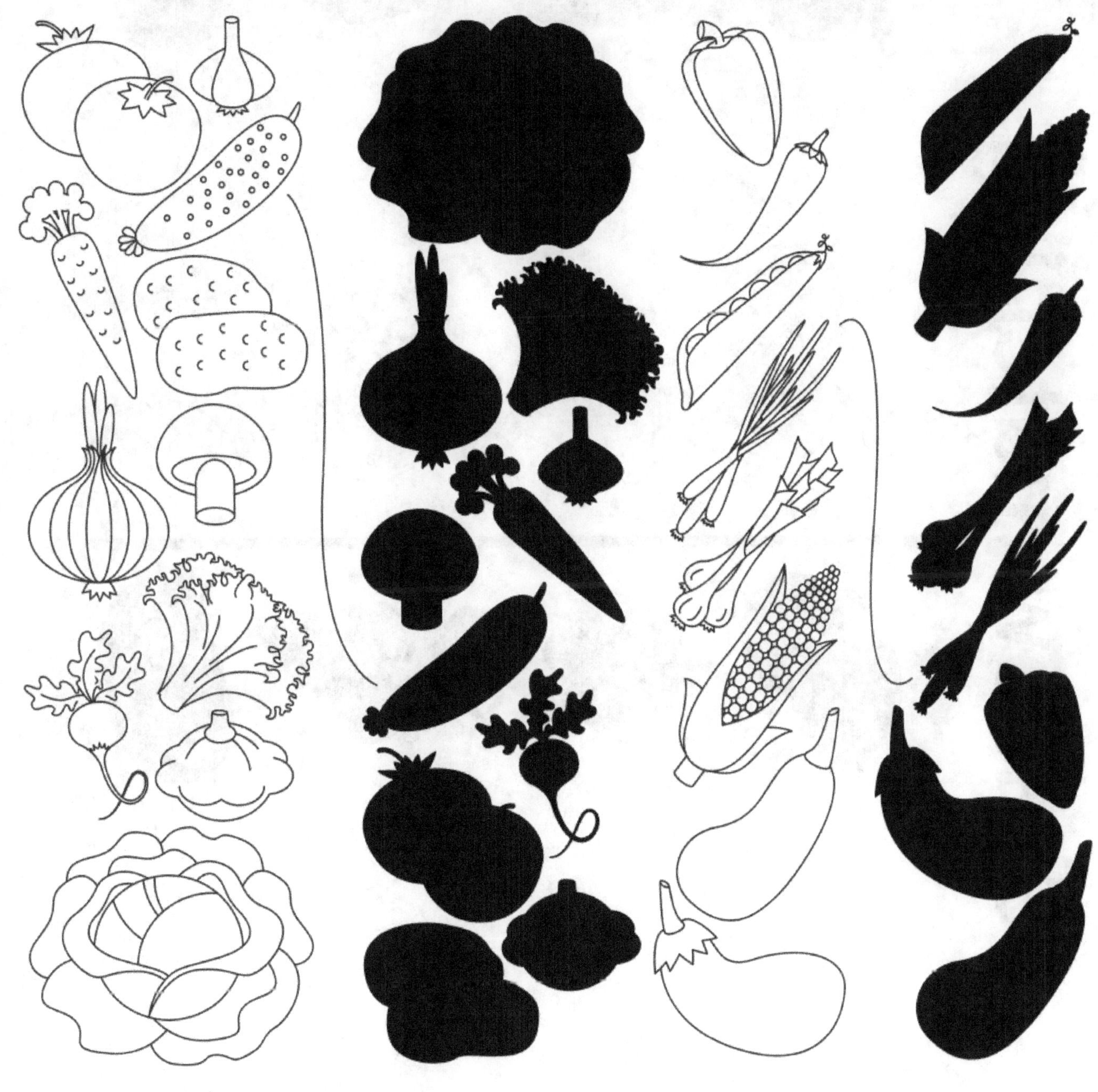

Shadow matching

Item hunt

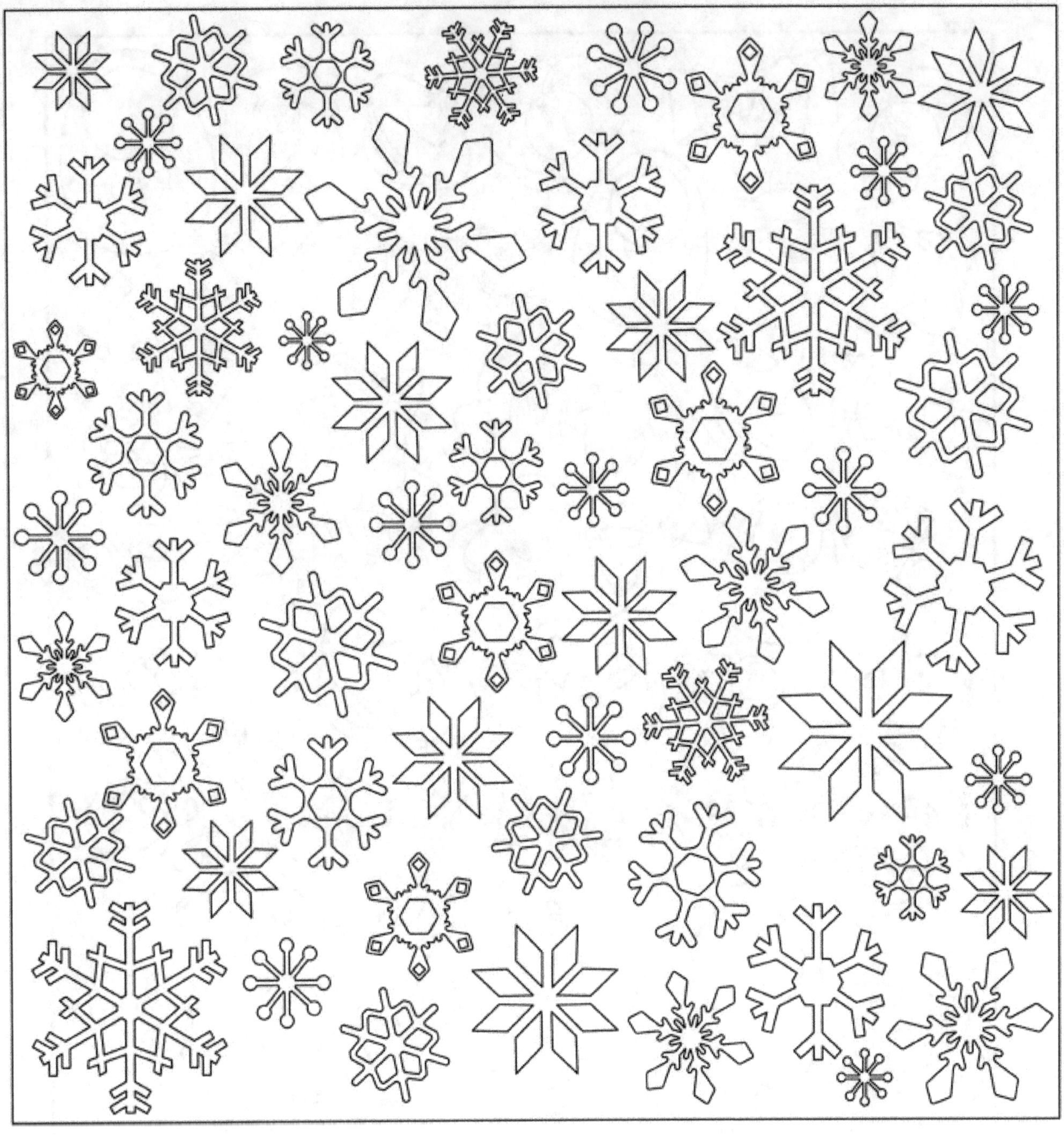

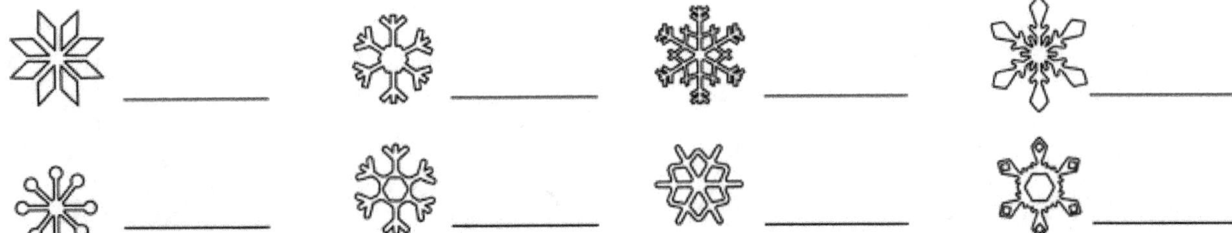

Item hunt

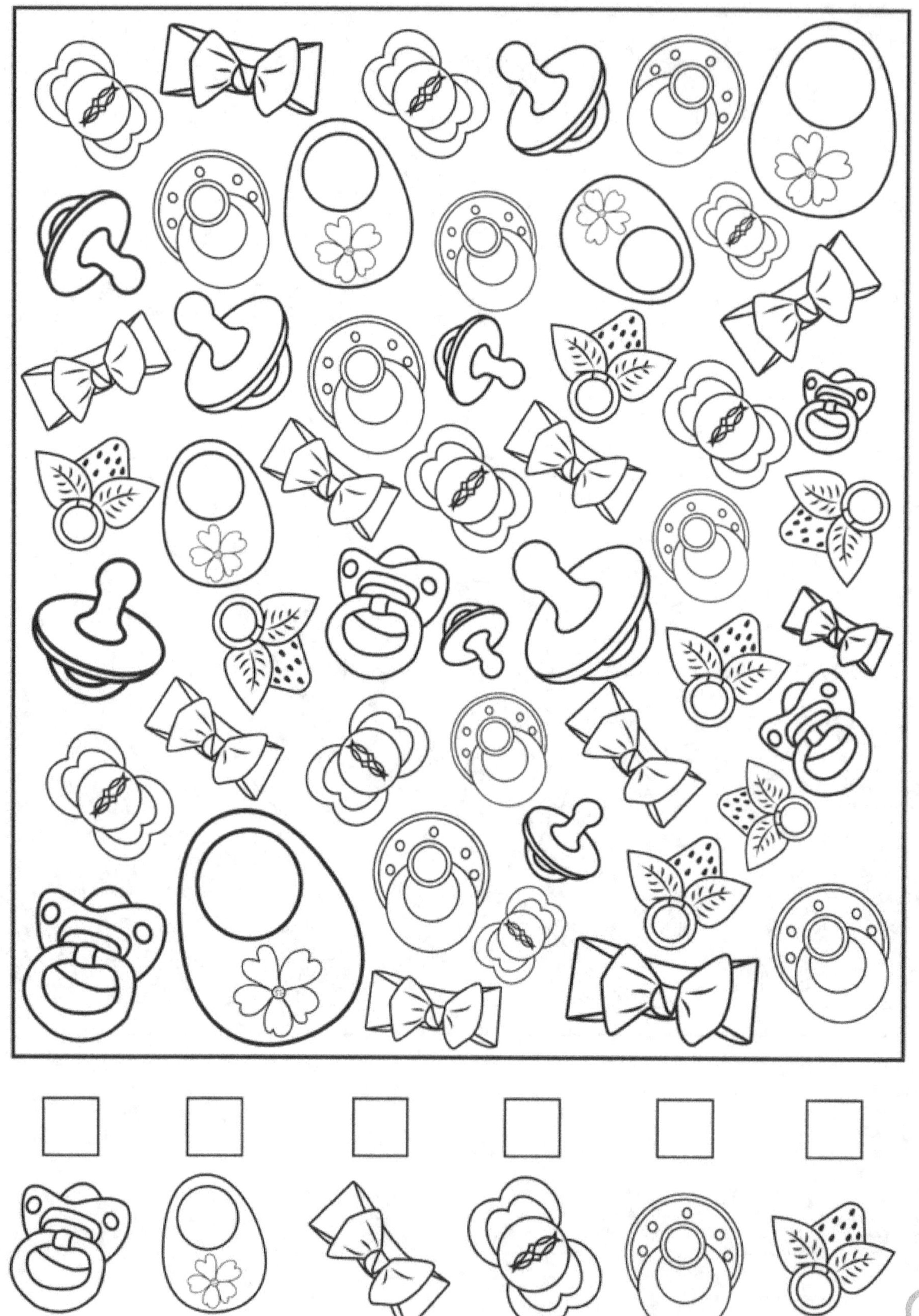

Item hunt

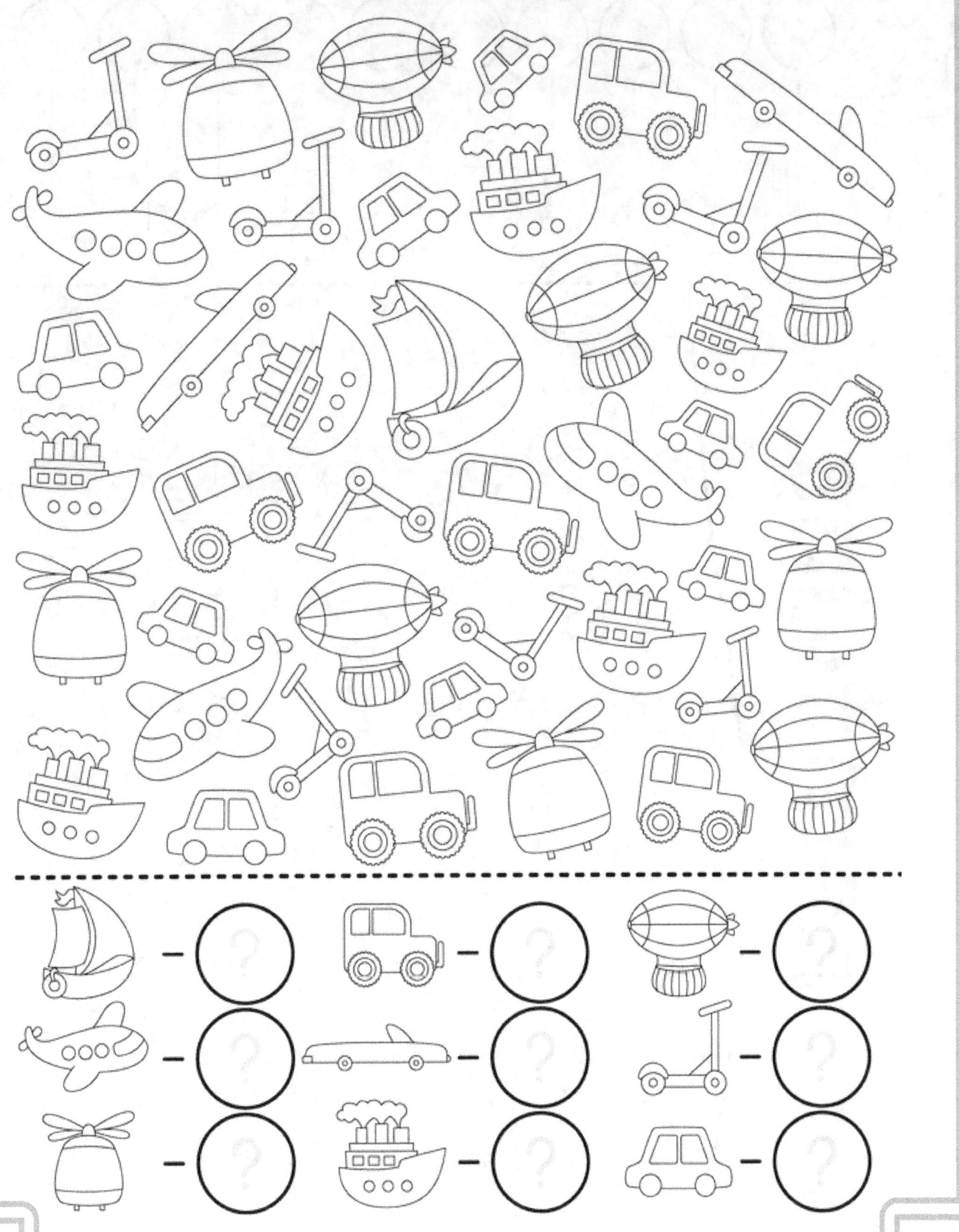

Item hunt

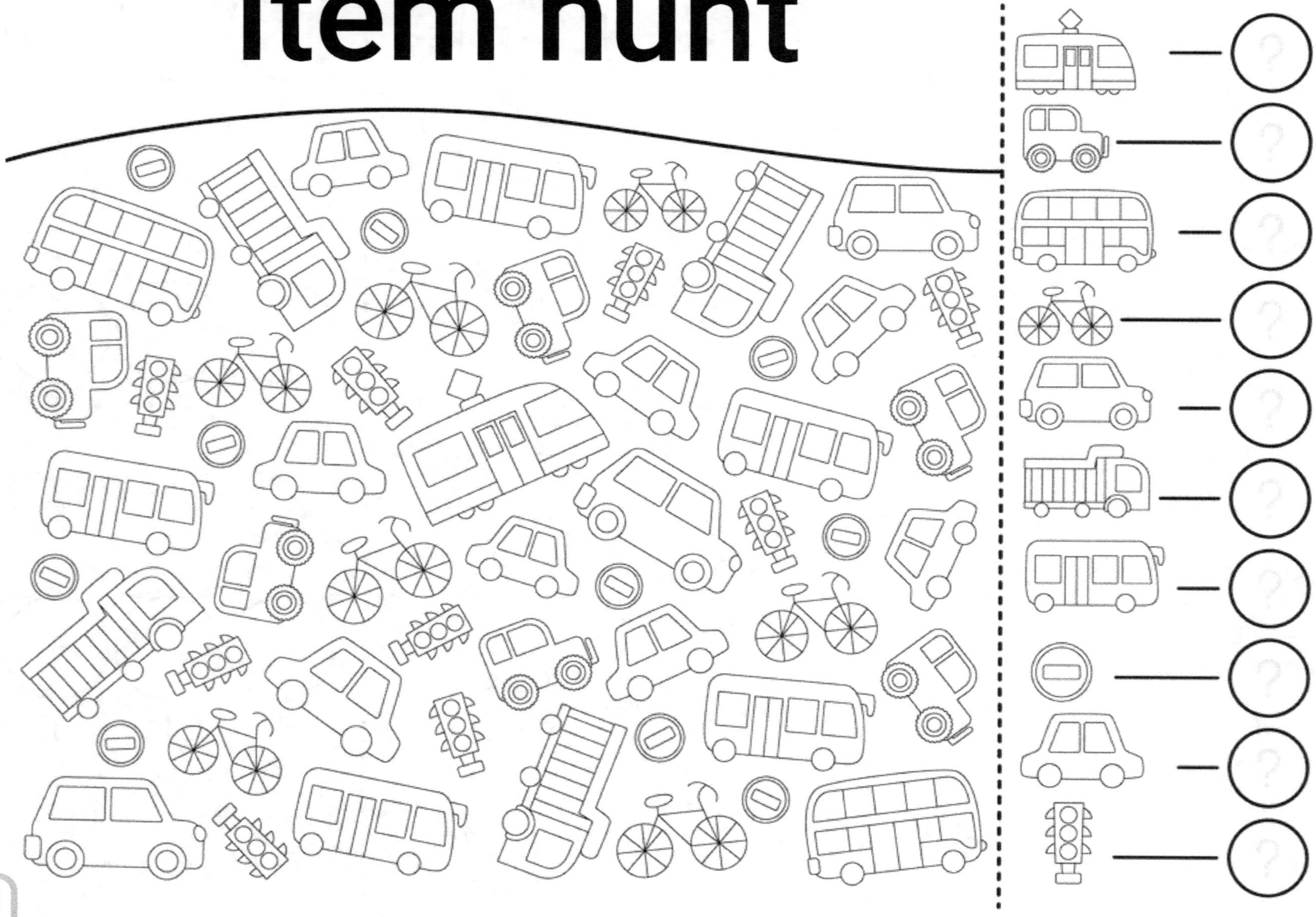

Item hunt

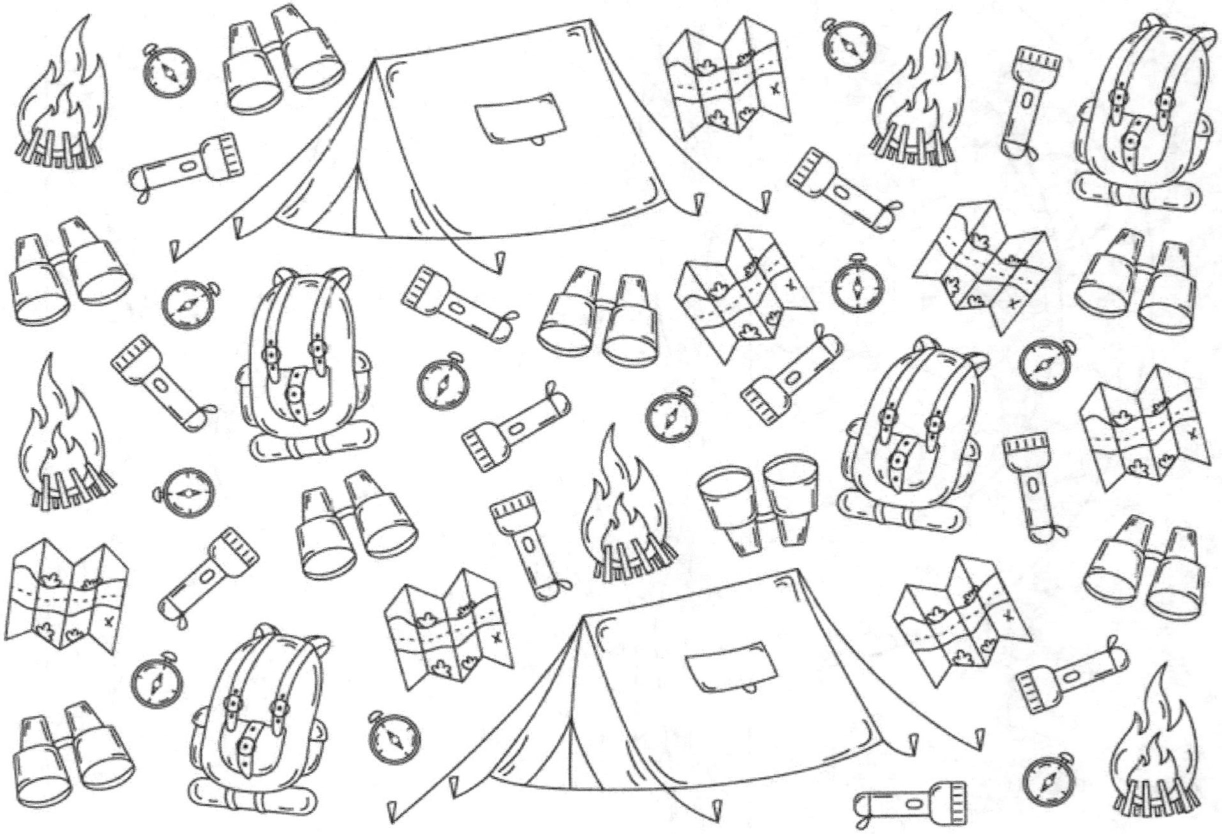

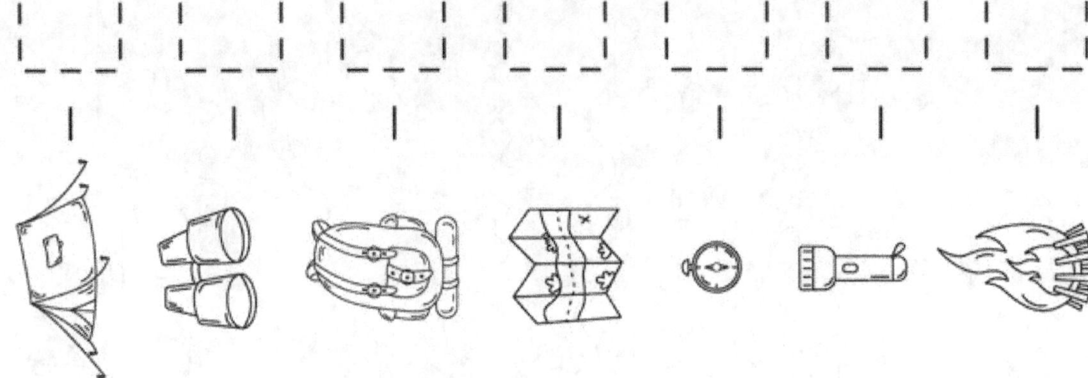

Coloring pages

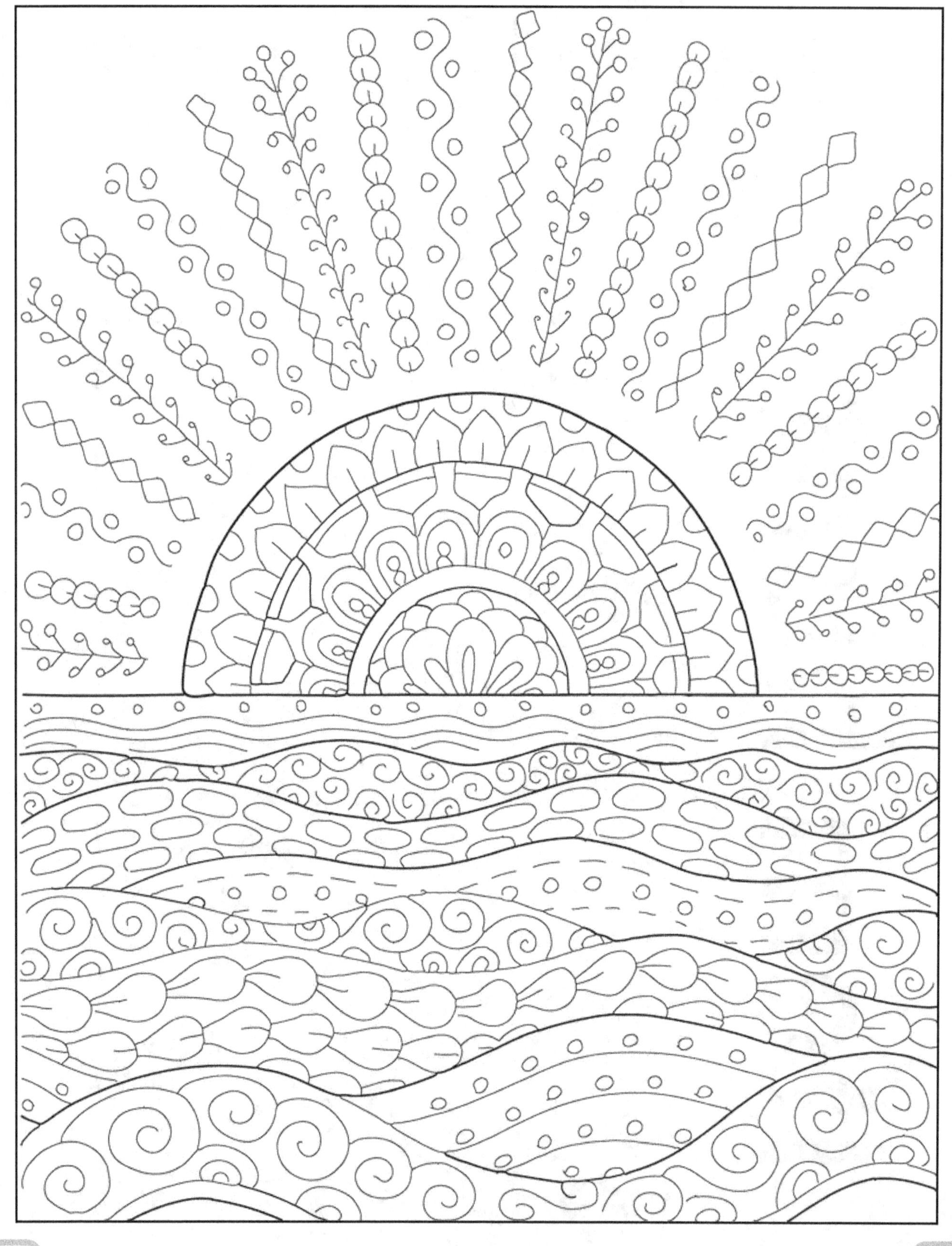

Coloring pages

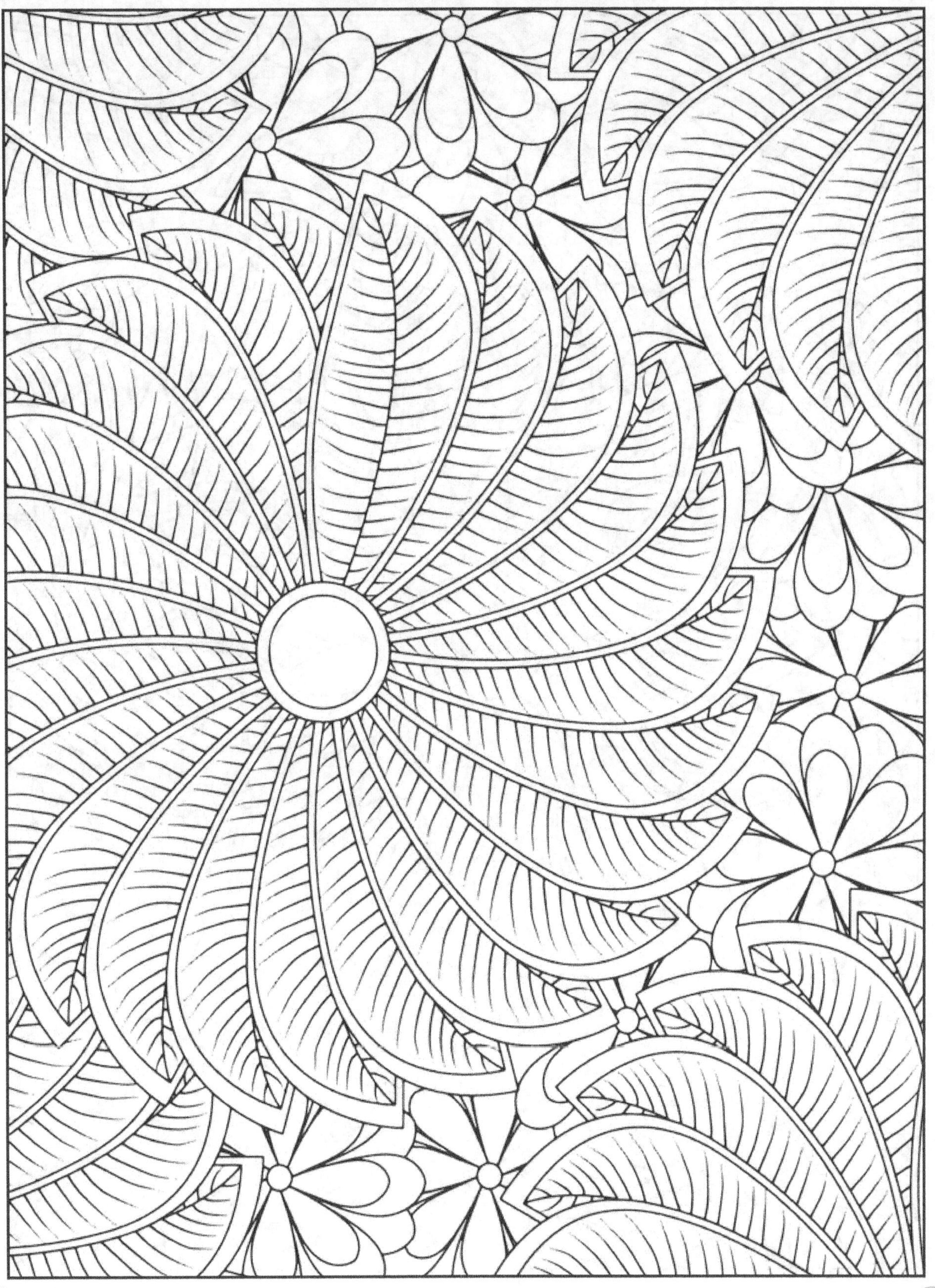

Coloring pages

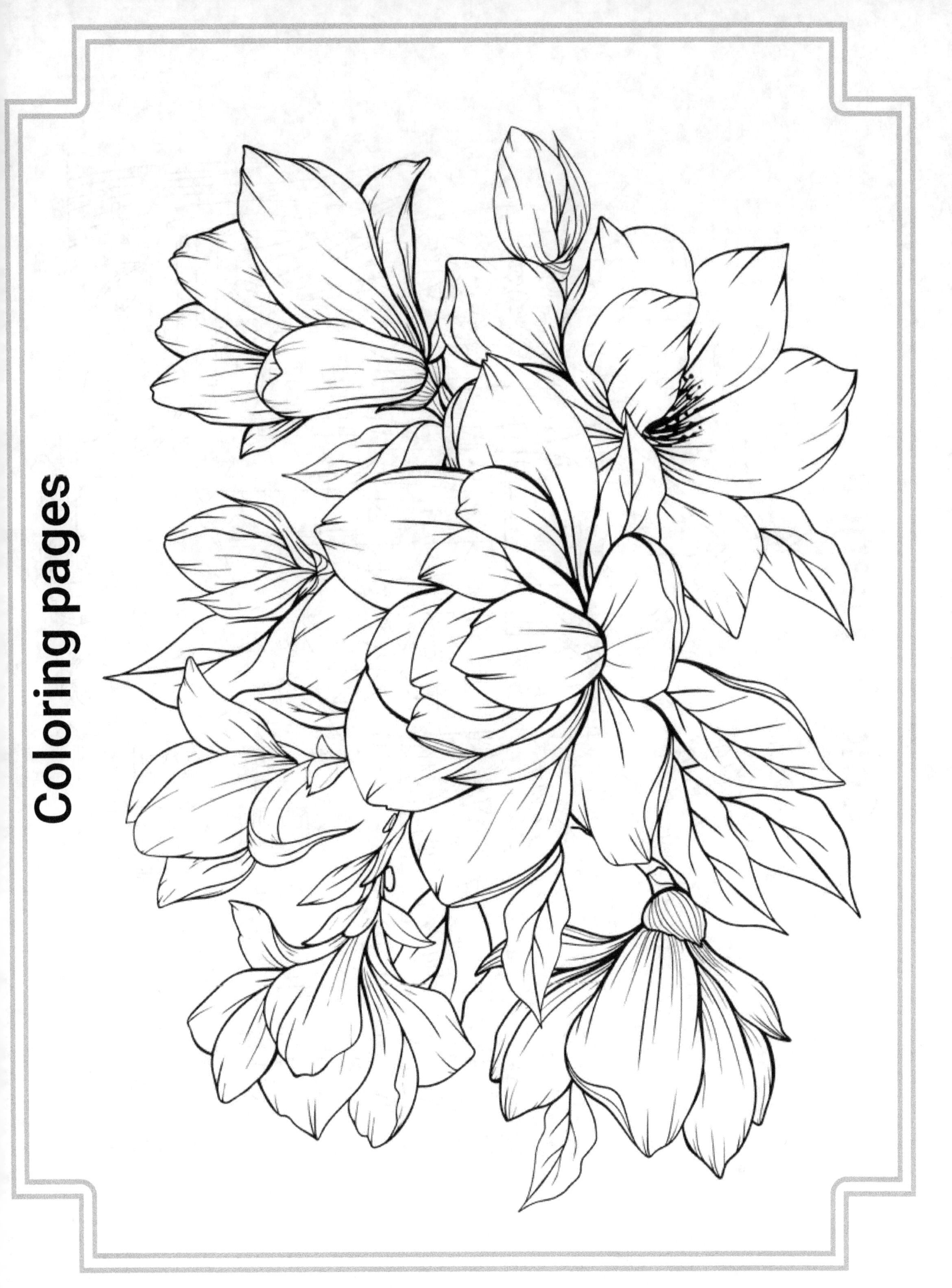
Coloring pages

Coloring pages

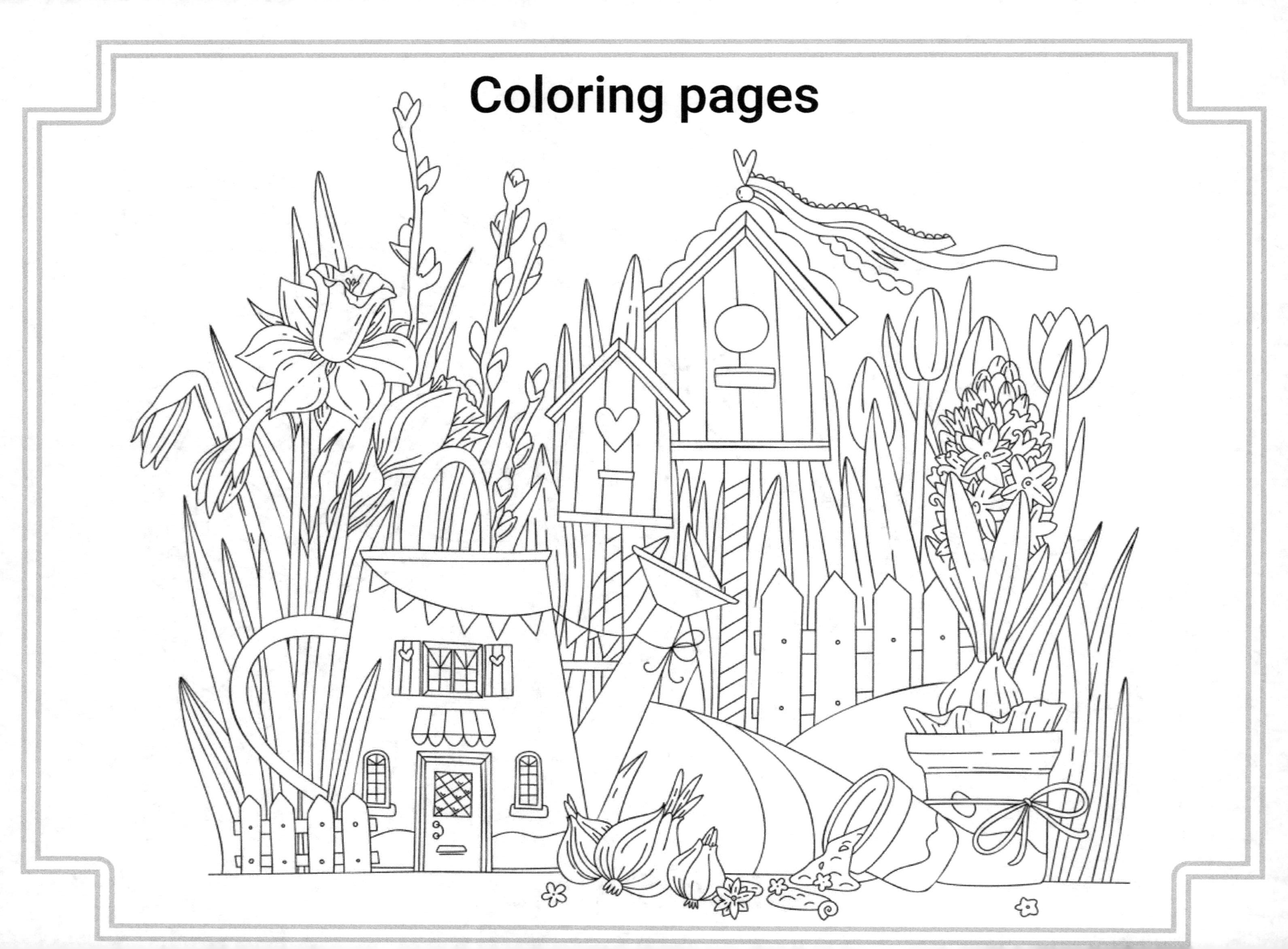

Coloring pages

Coloring pages

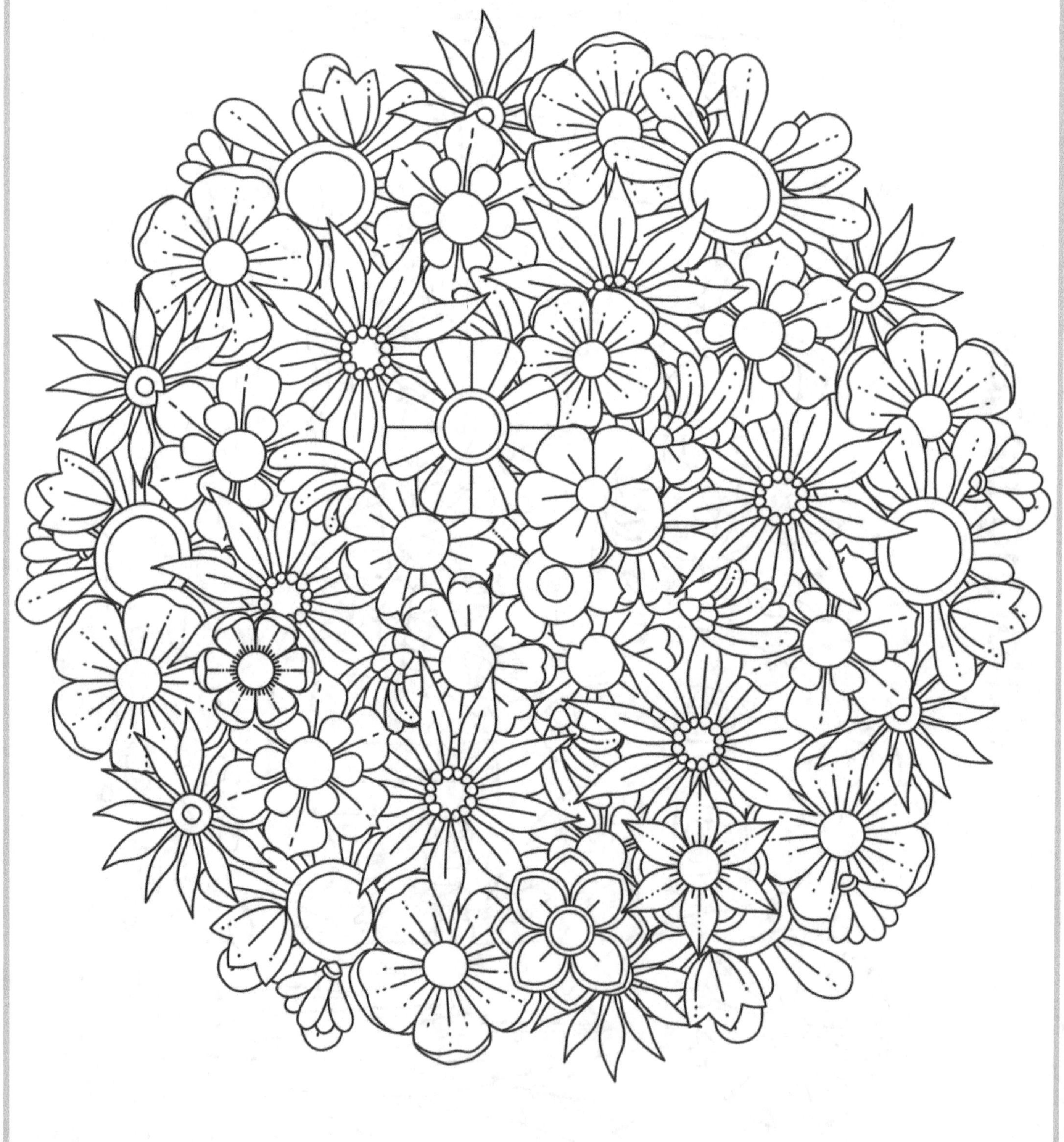

Coloring pages

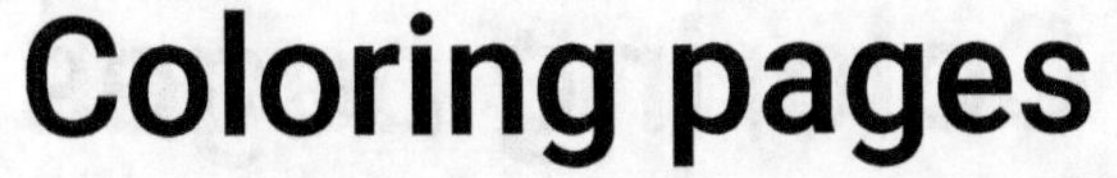

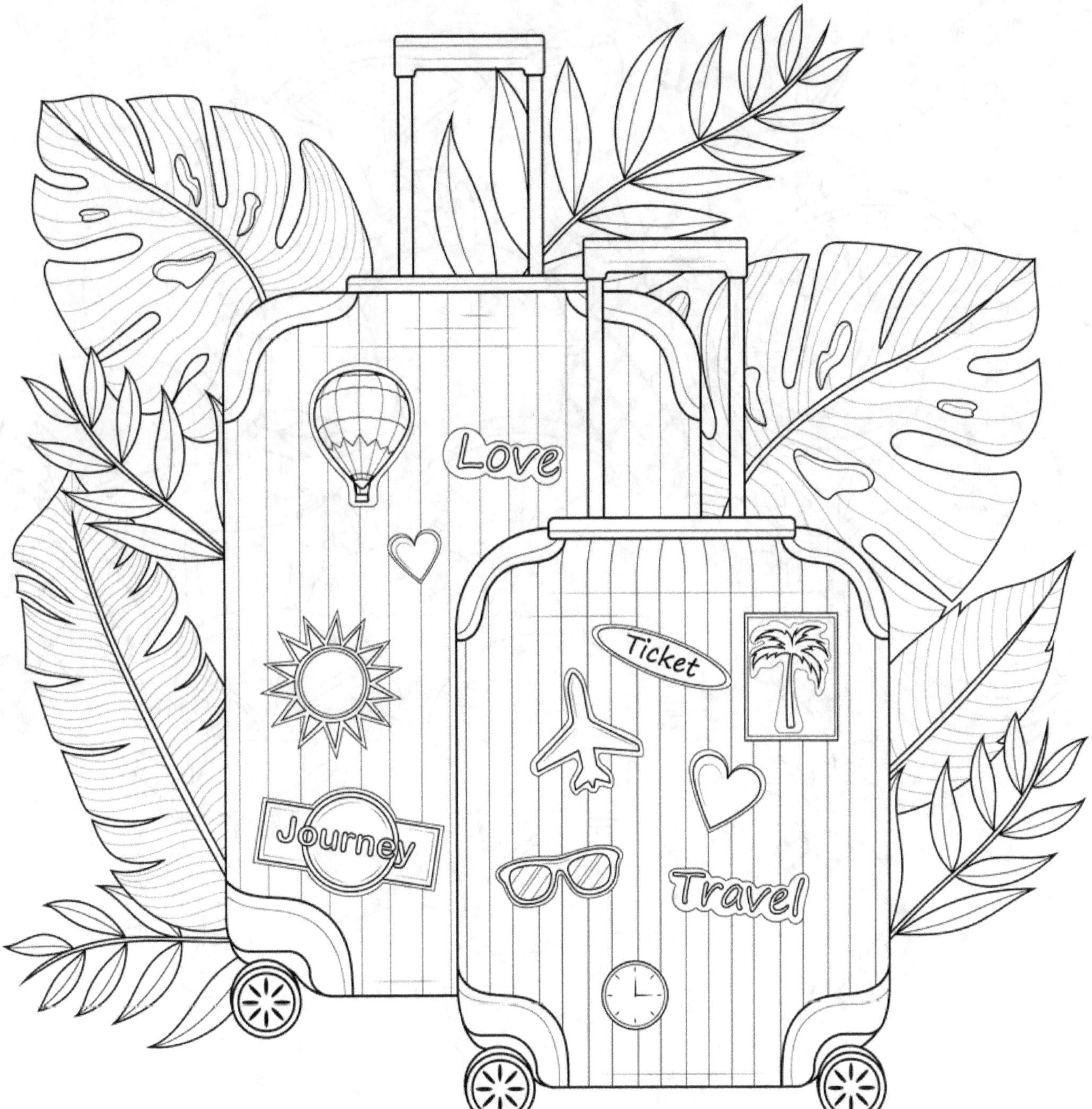

Coloring pages

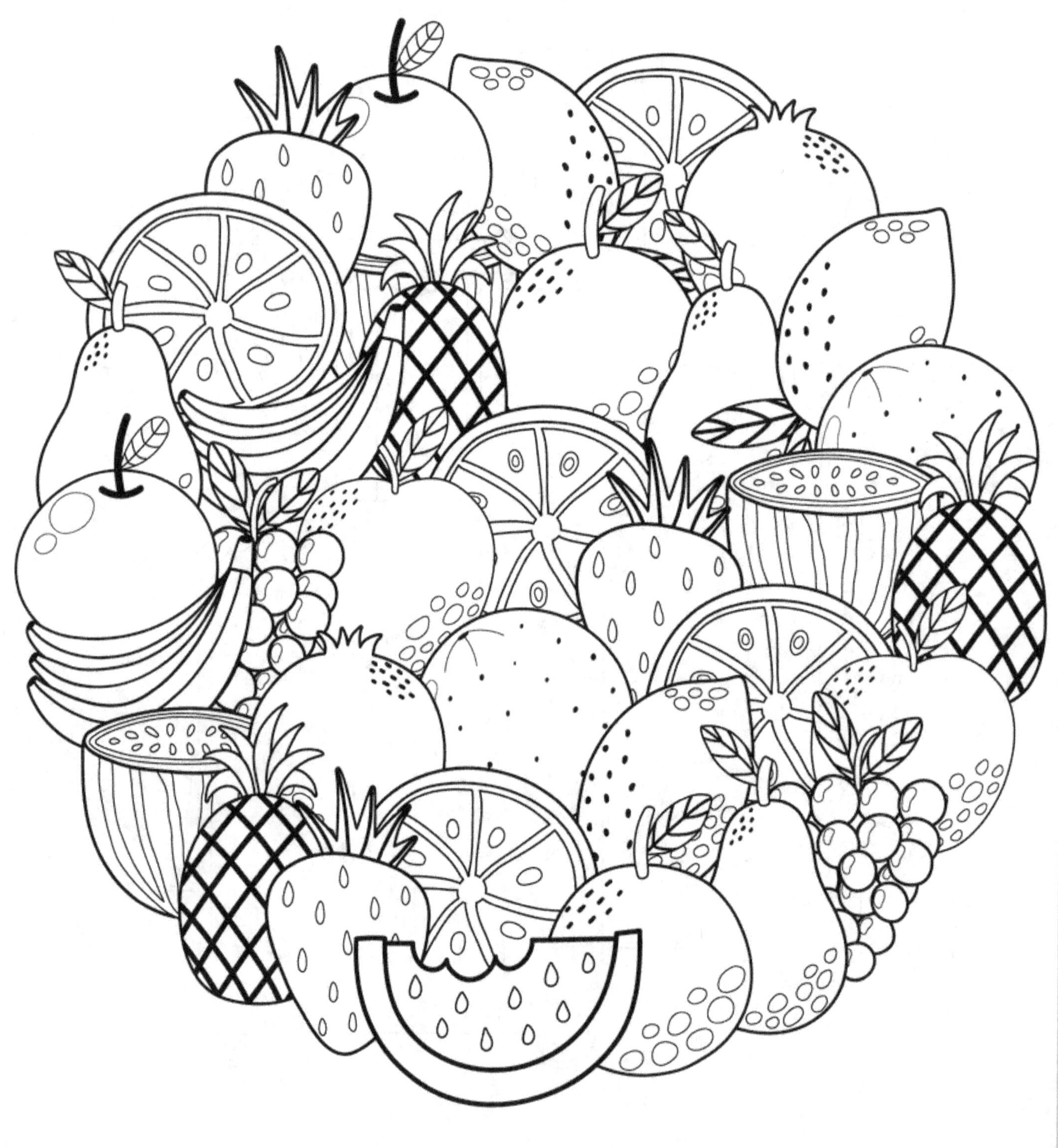

Coloring pages

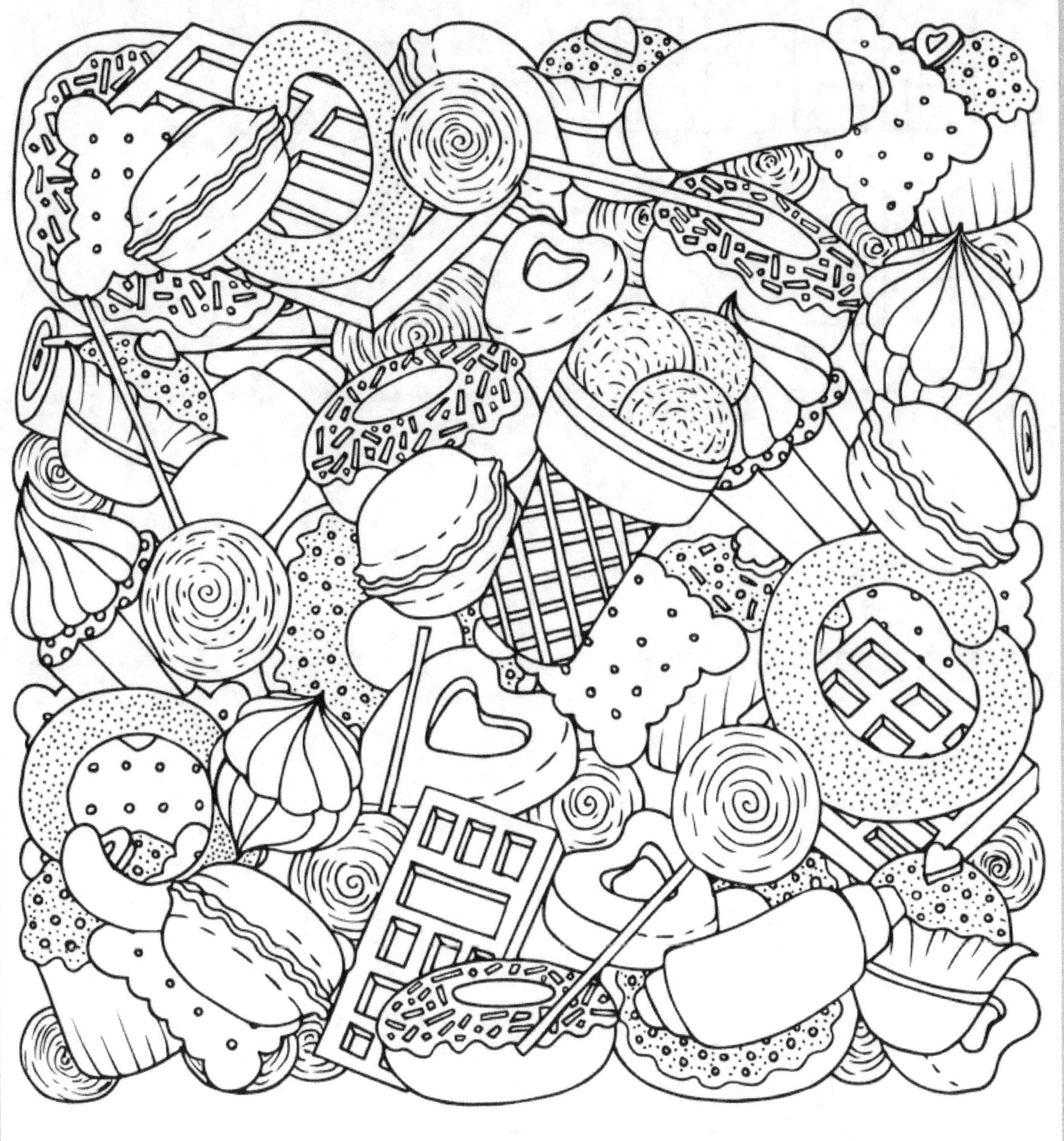

Continue the pattern

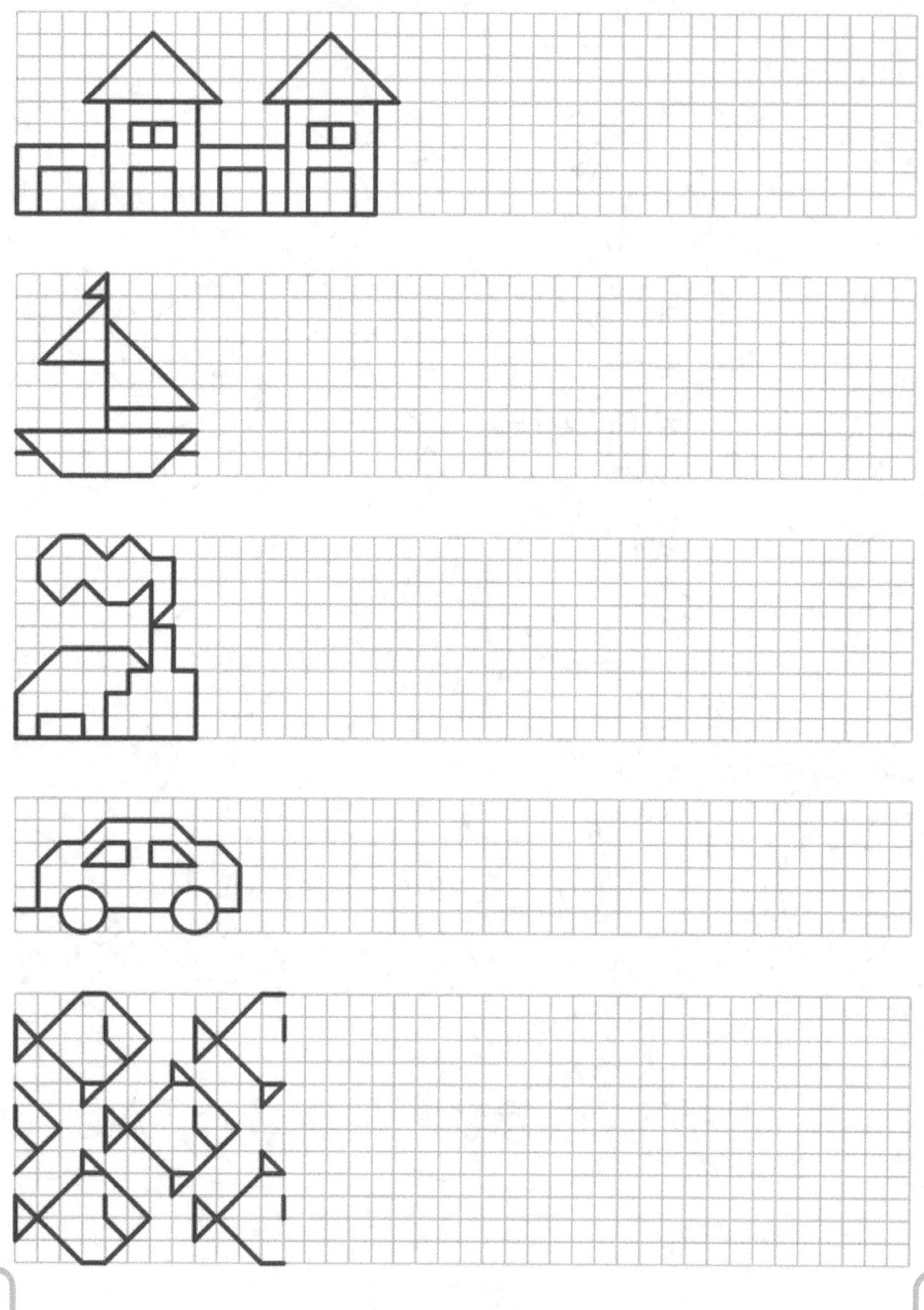

Continue the pattern

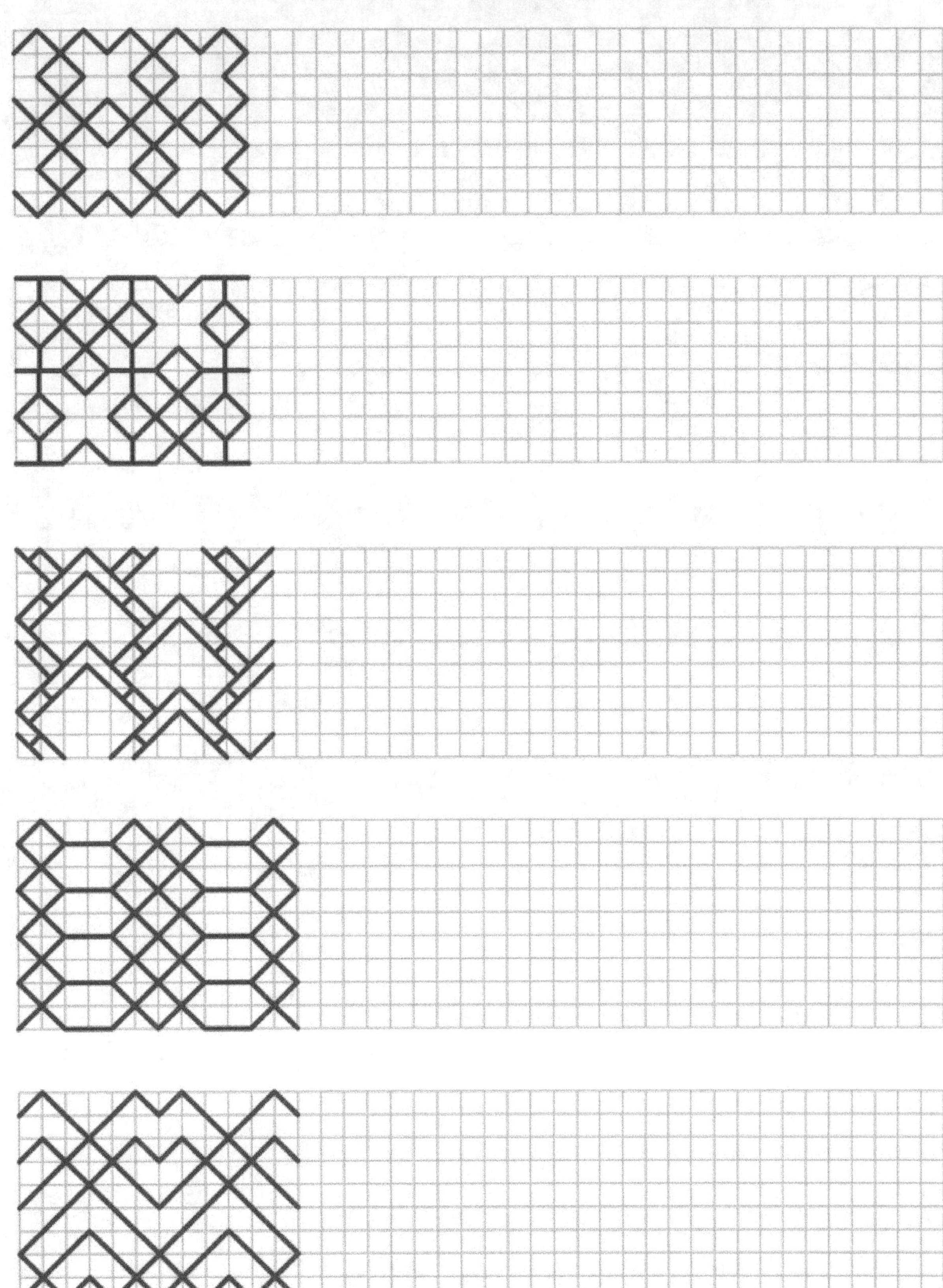

Continue the pattern

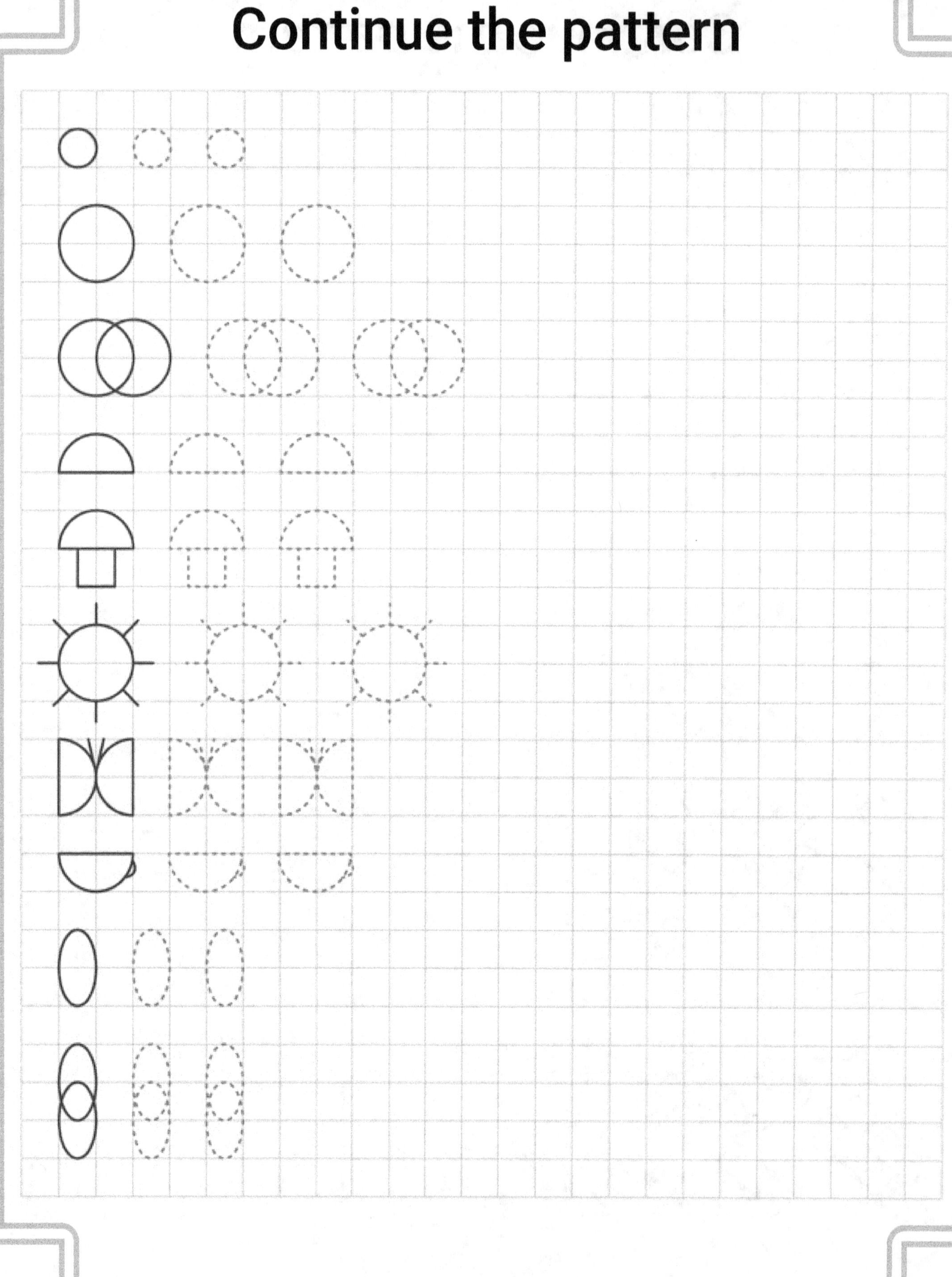

Eye-hand coordination

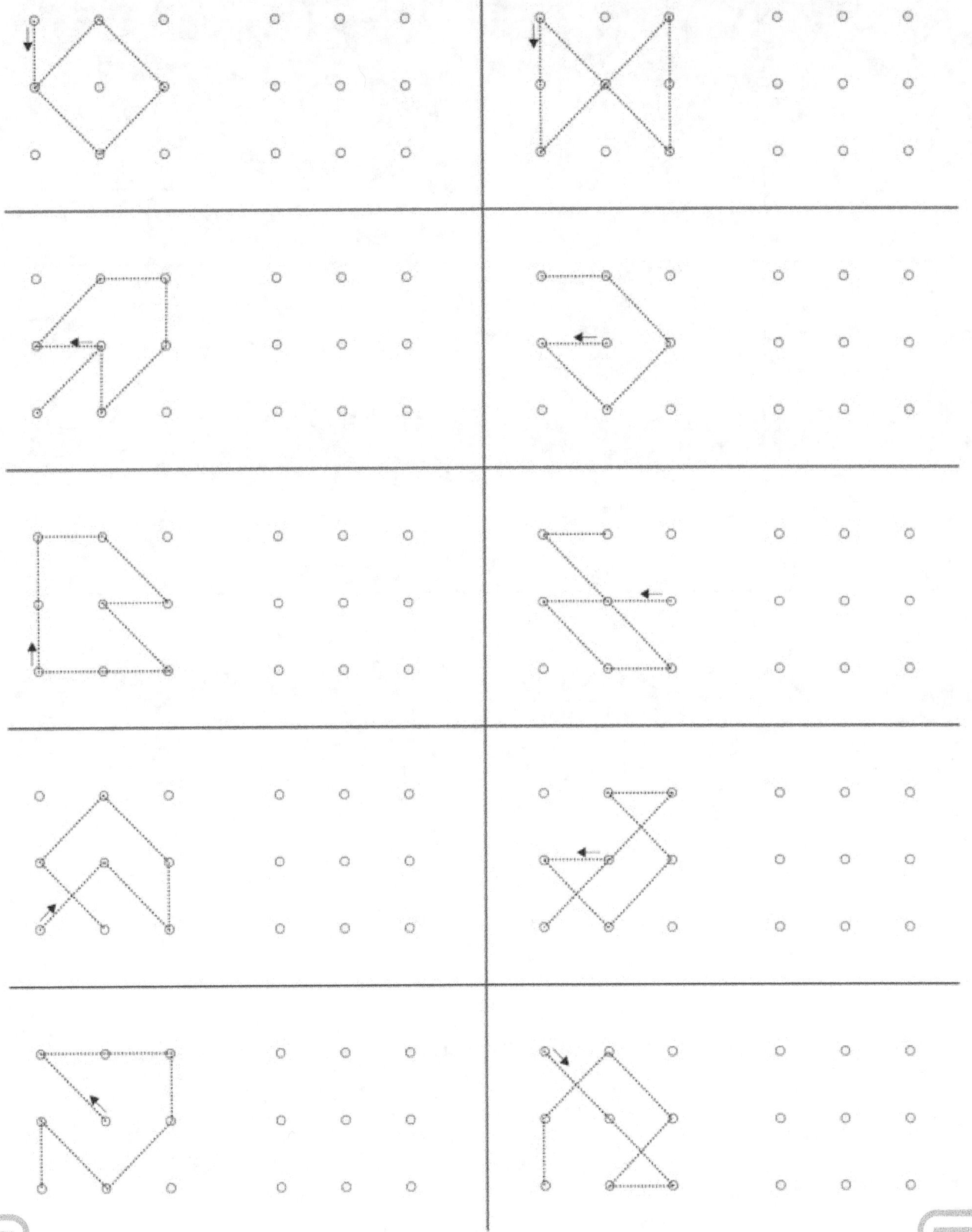

Eye-hand coordination

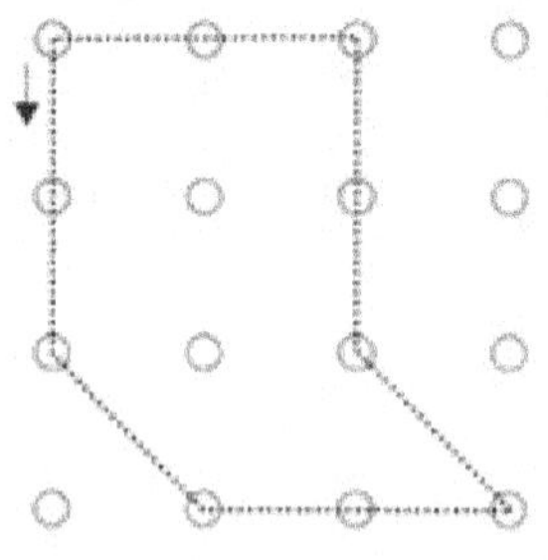 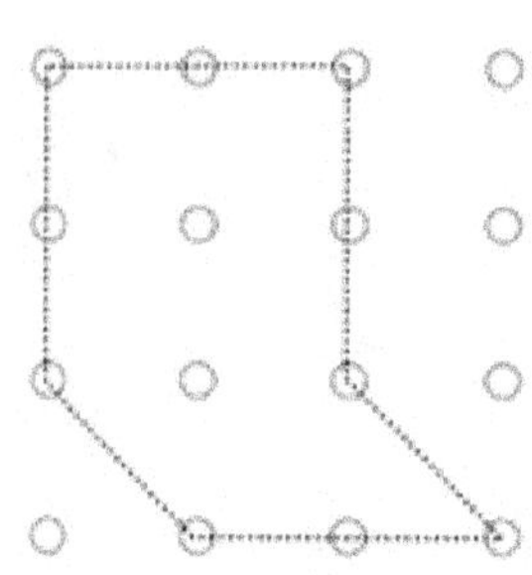 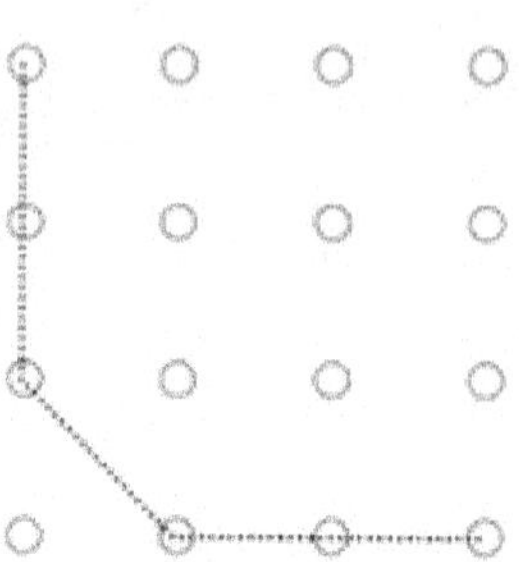

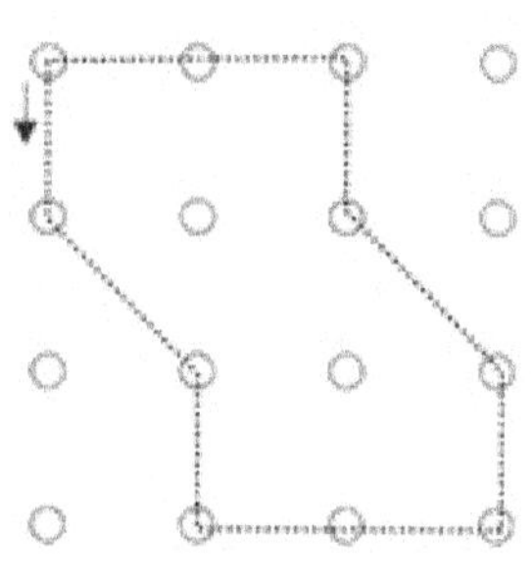 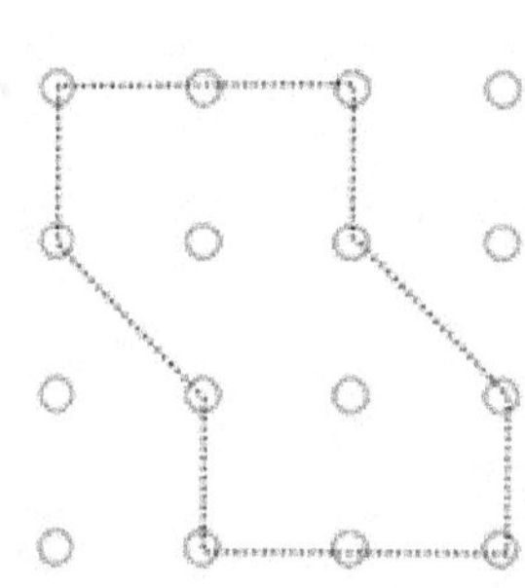 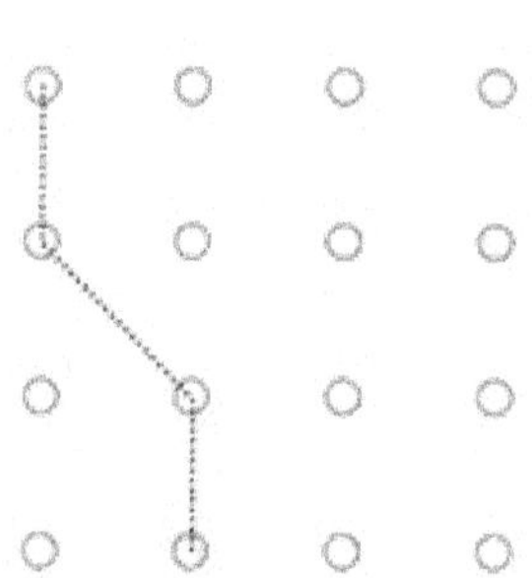

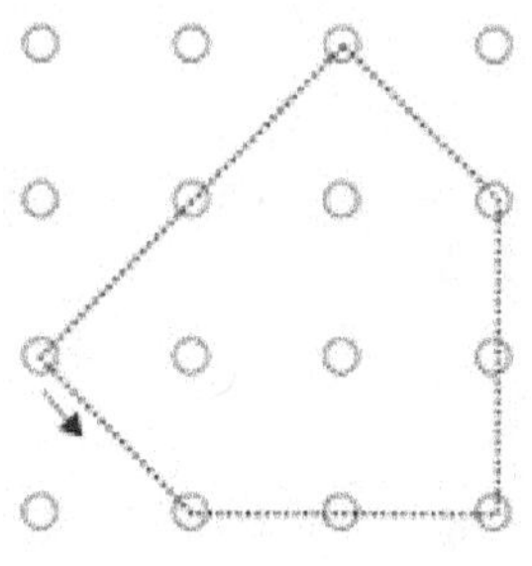 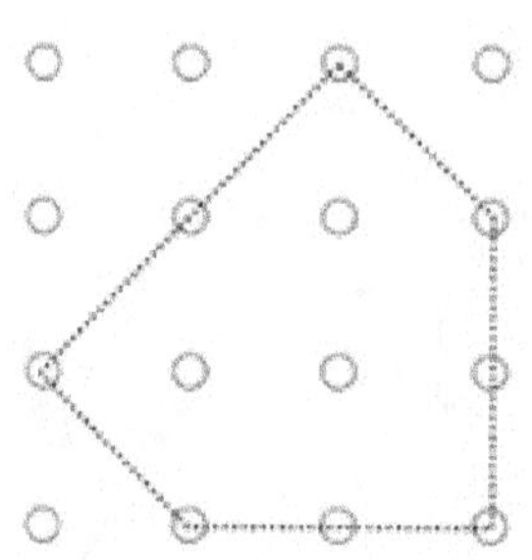 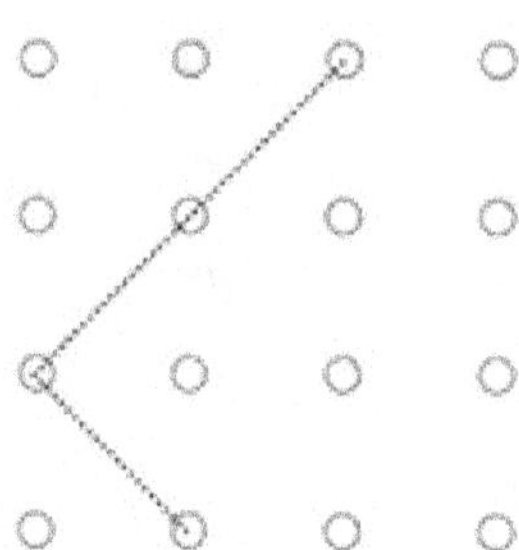

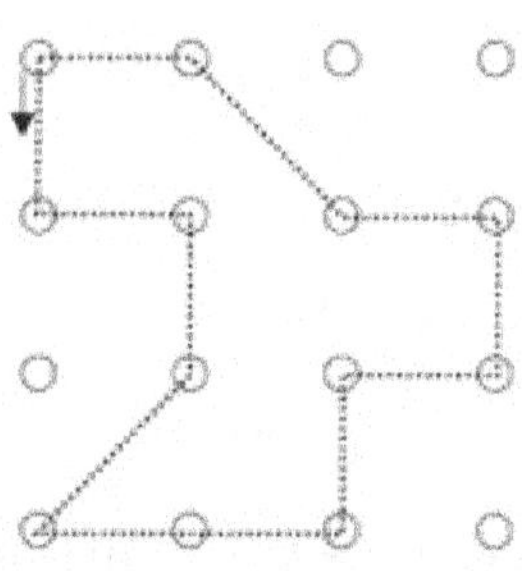 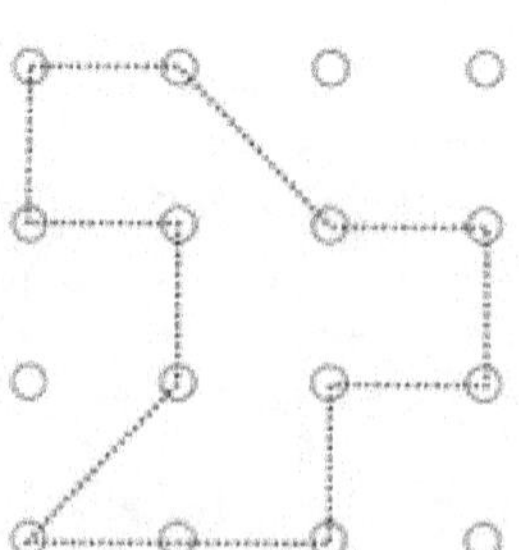 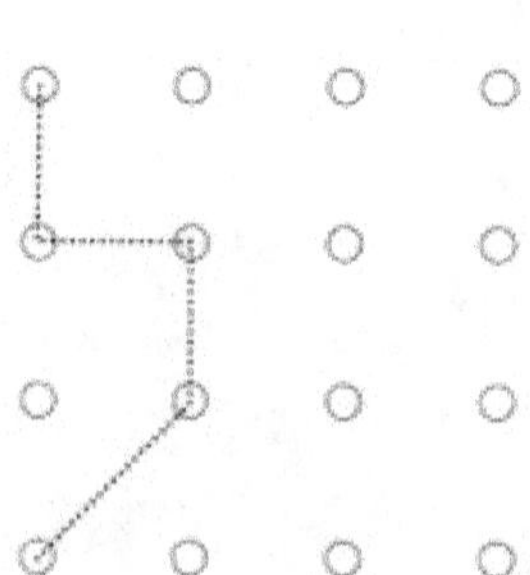

Eye-hand coordination

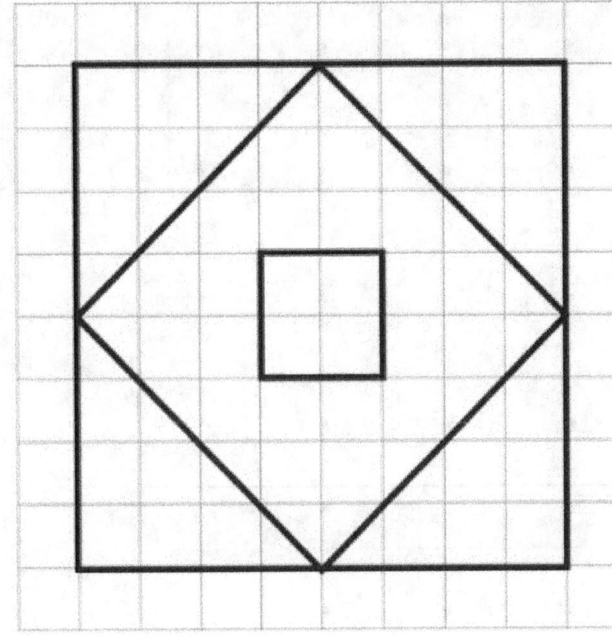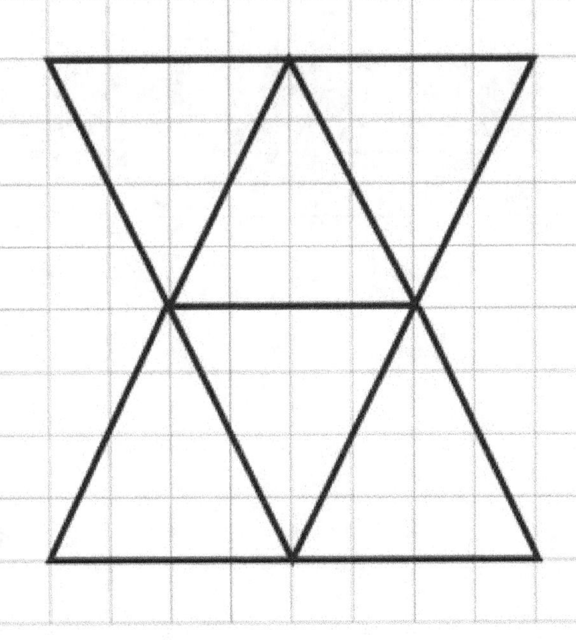

Eye-hand coordination

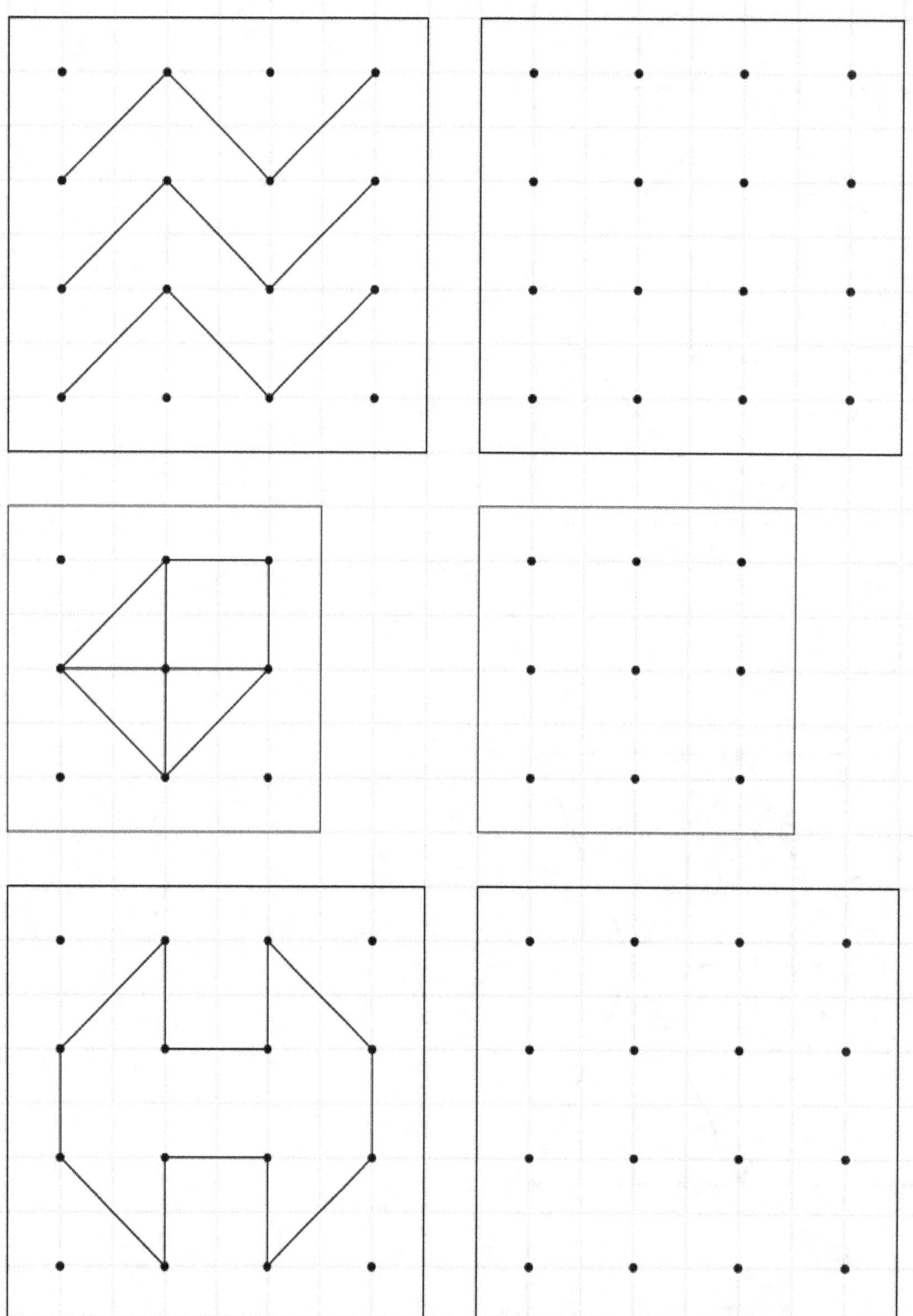

Eye-hand coordination

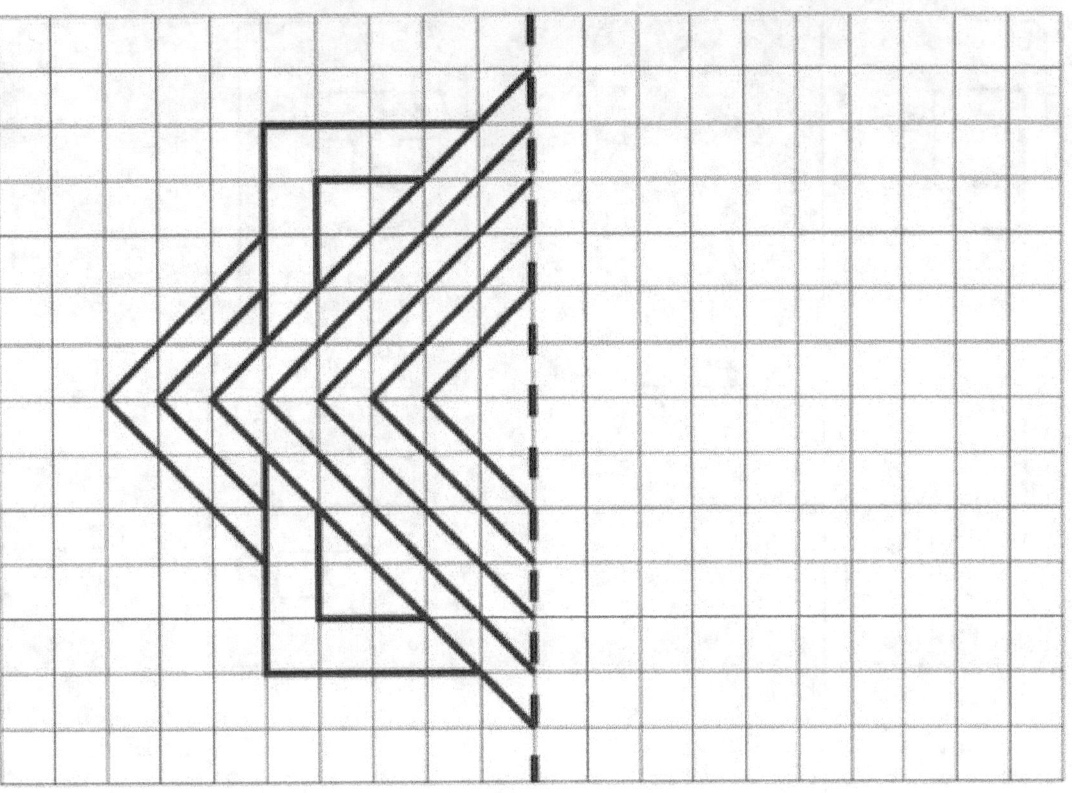

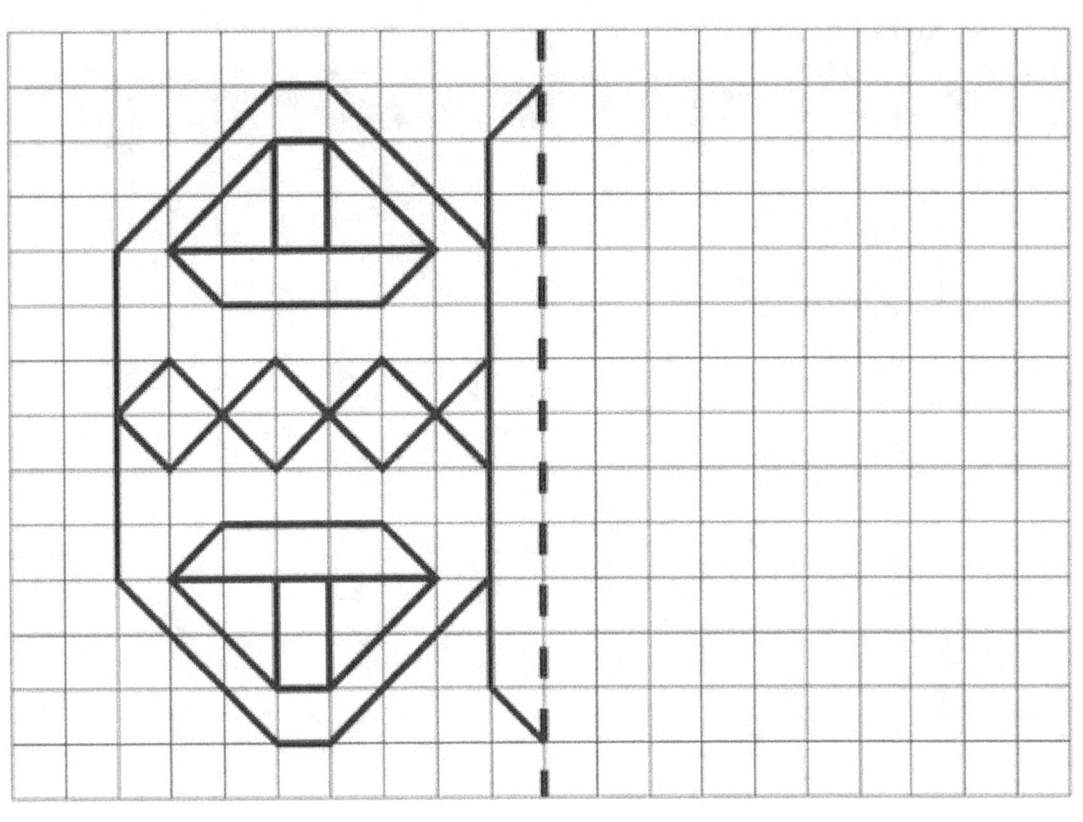

Eye-hand coordination

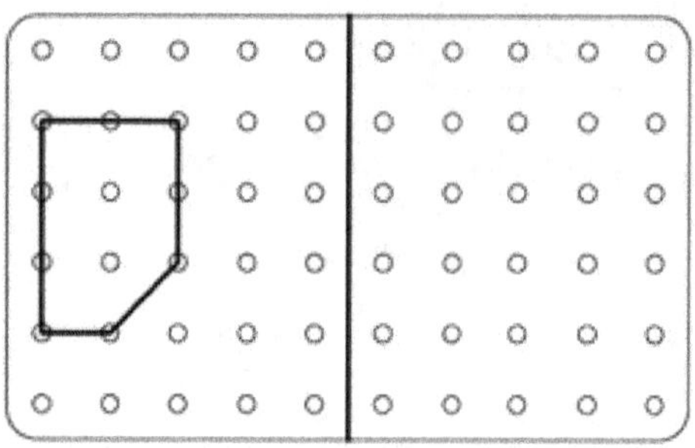 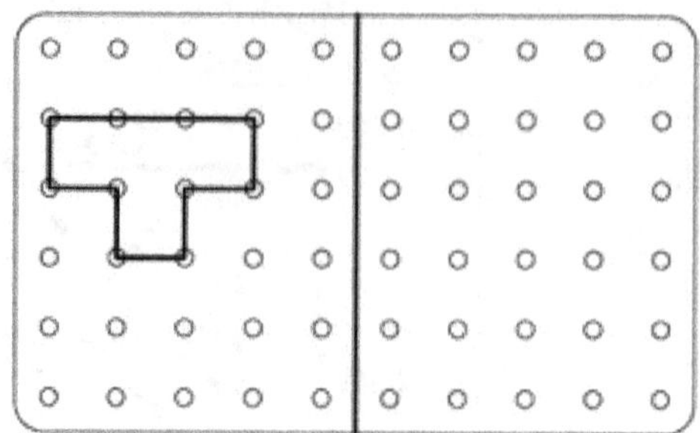

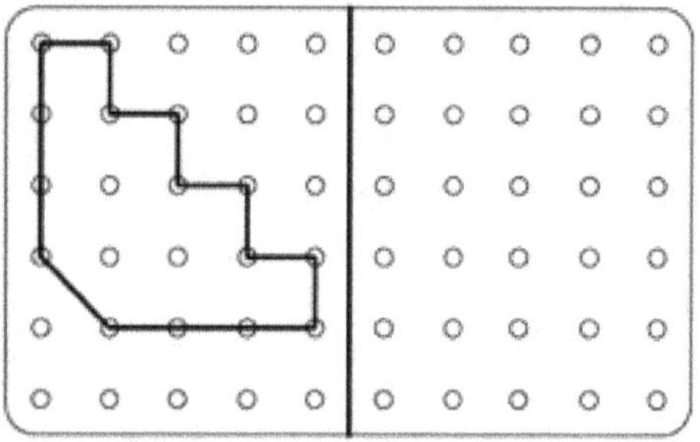 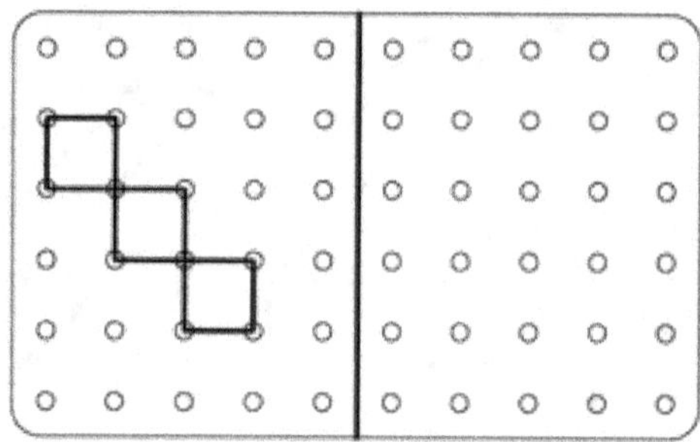

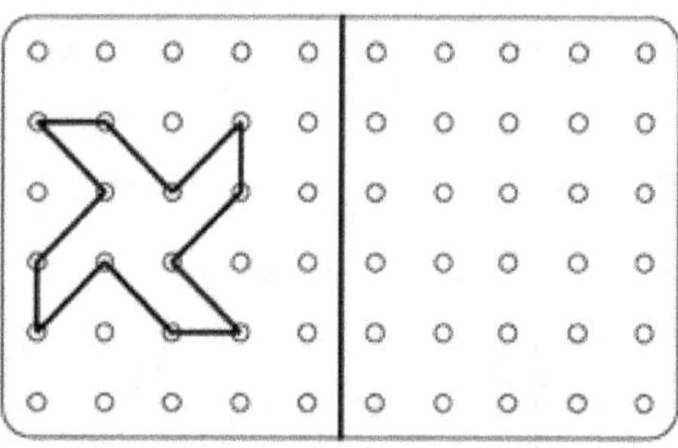 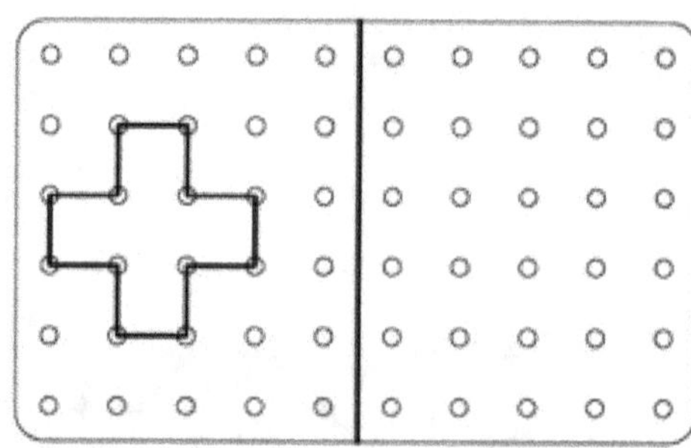

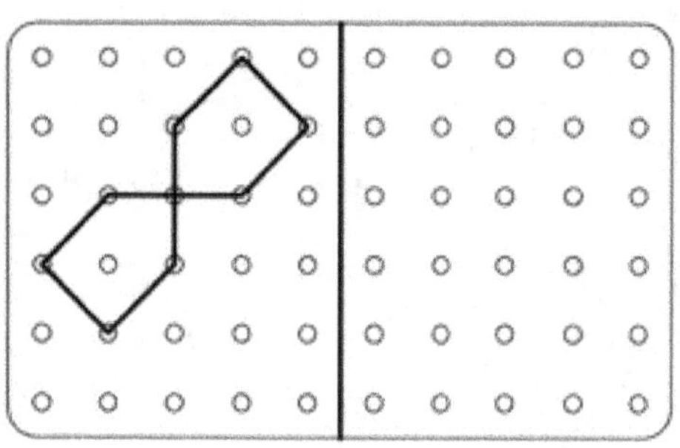 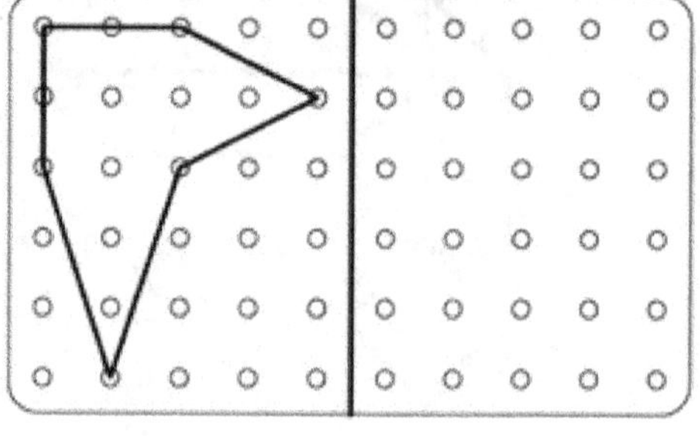

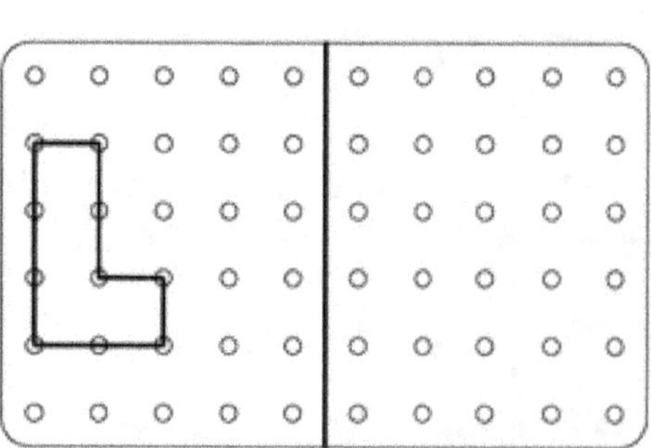 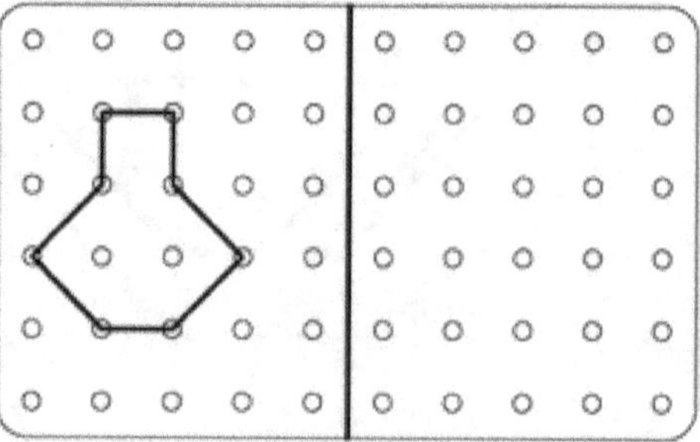

Find the ten differences between the two pictures.

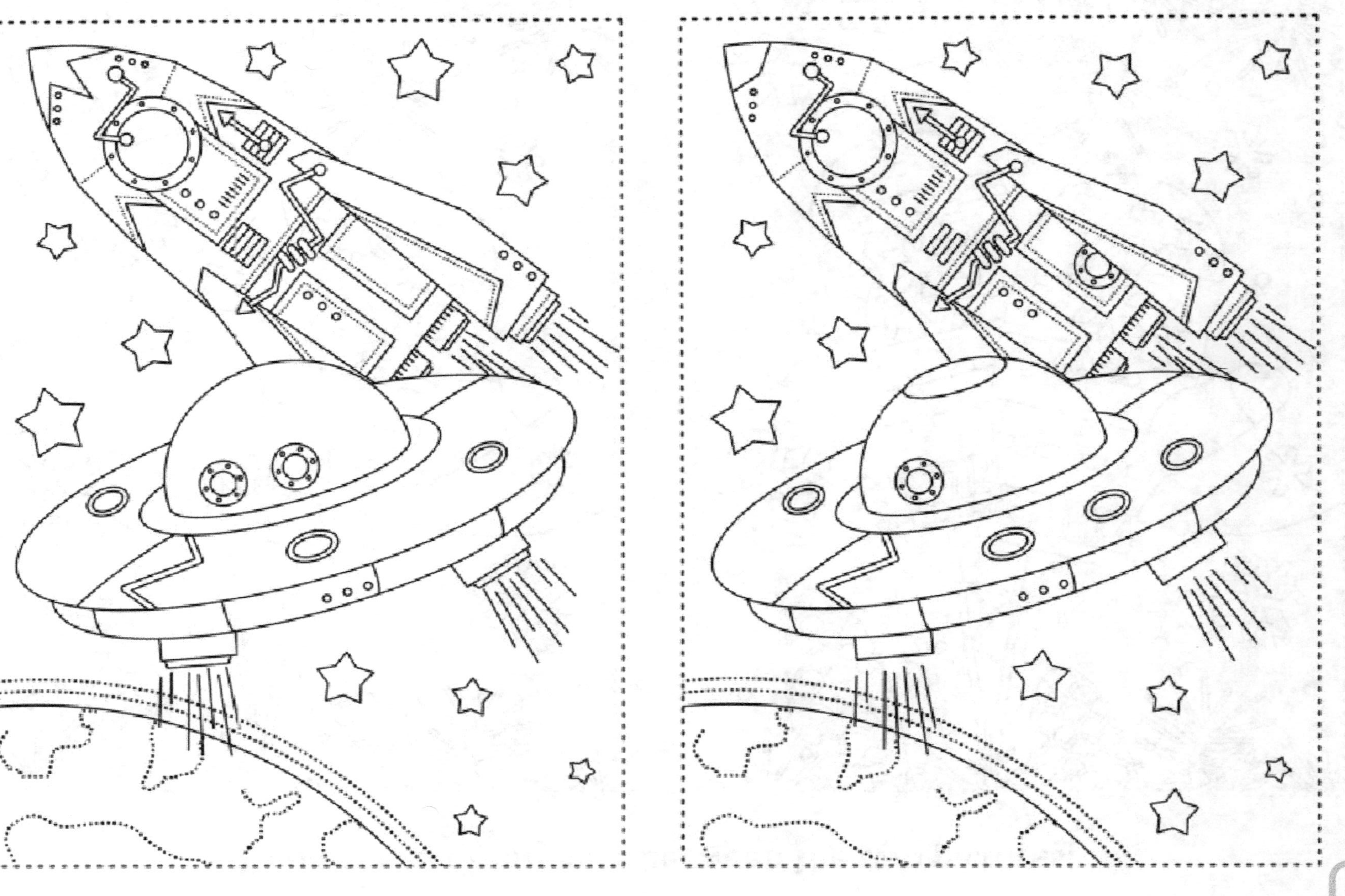

Find the ten differences between the two pictures.

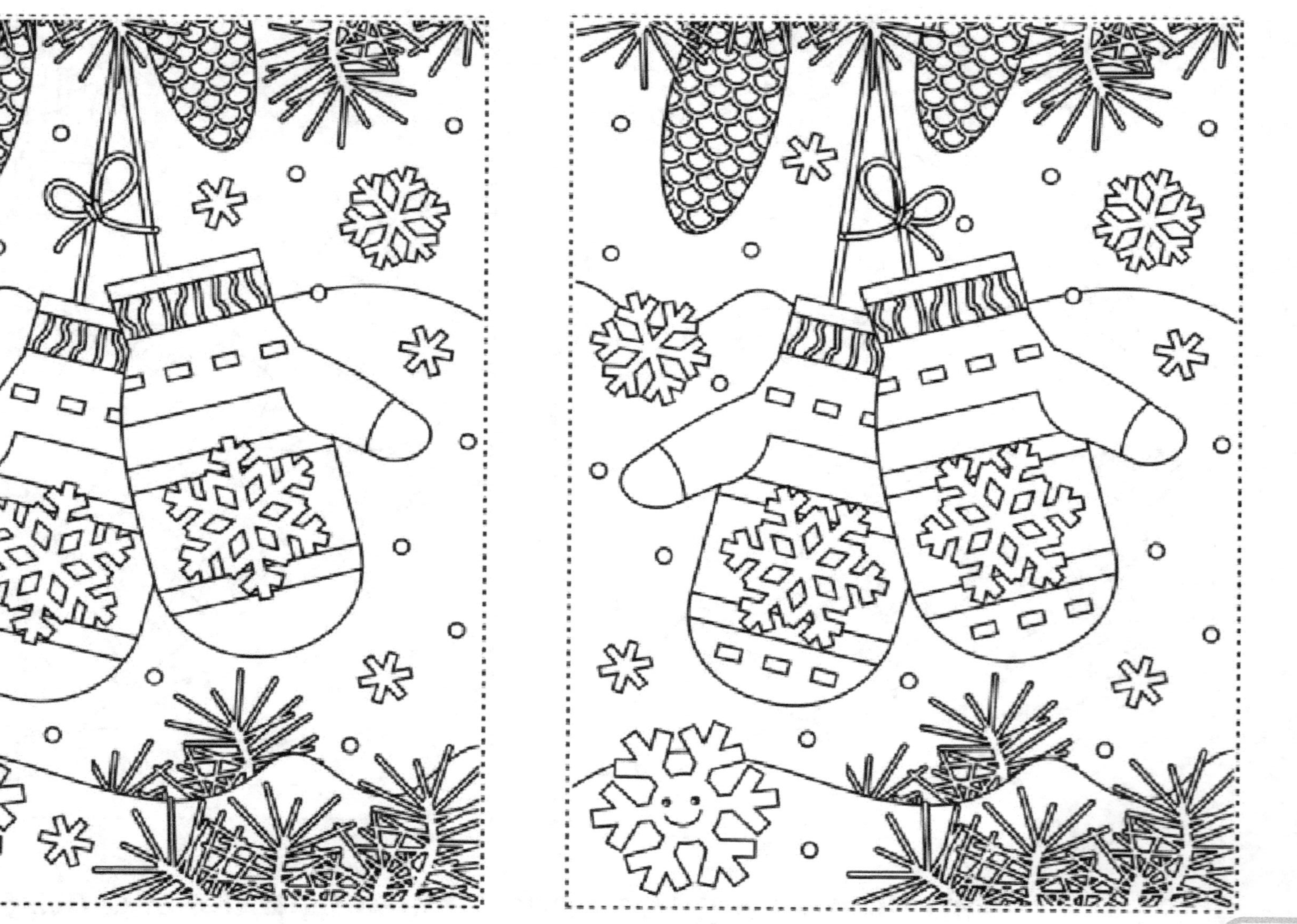

Find the ten differences between the two pictures.

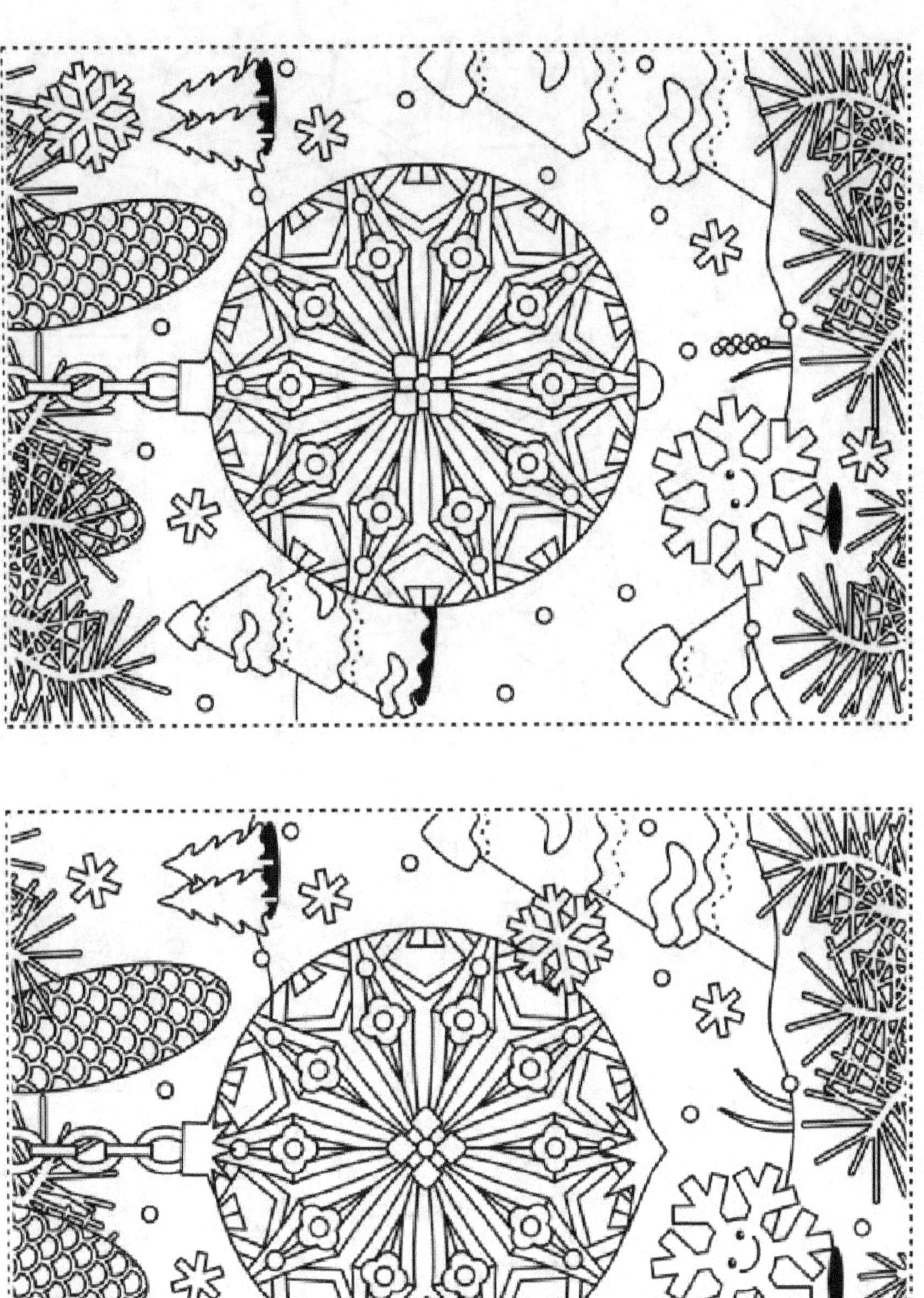

Find 10 differences.

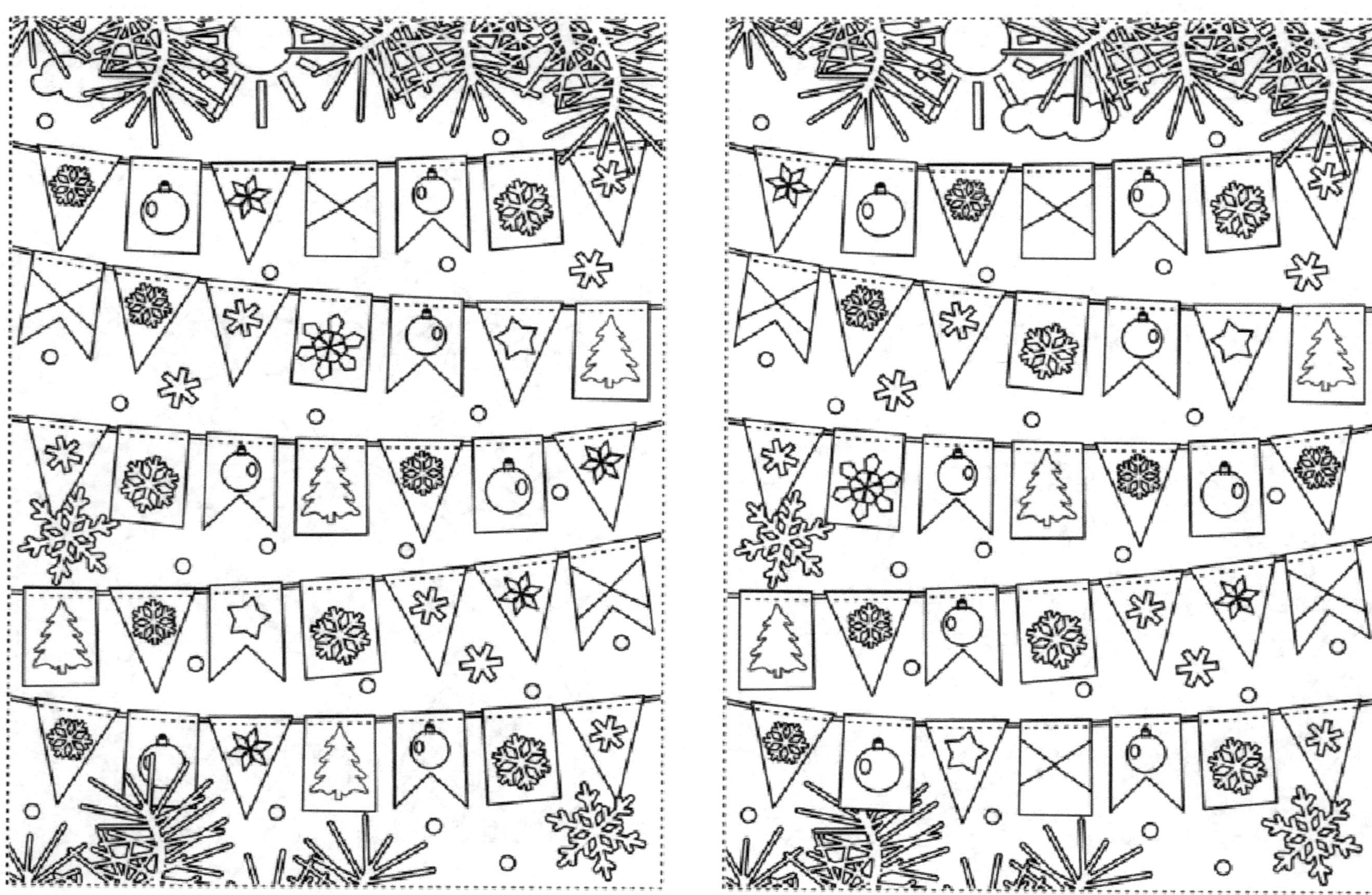

Find 10 differences.

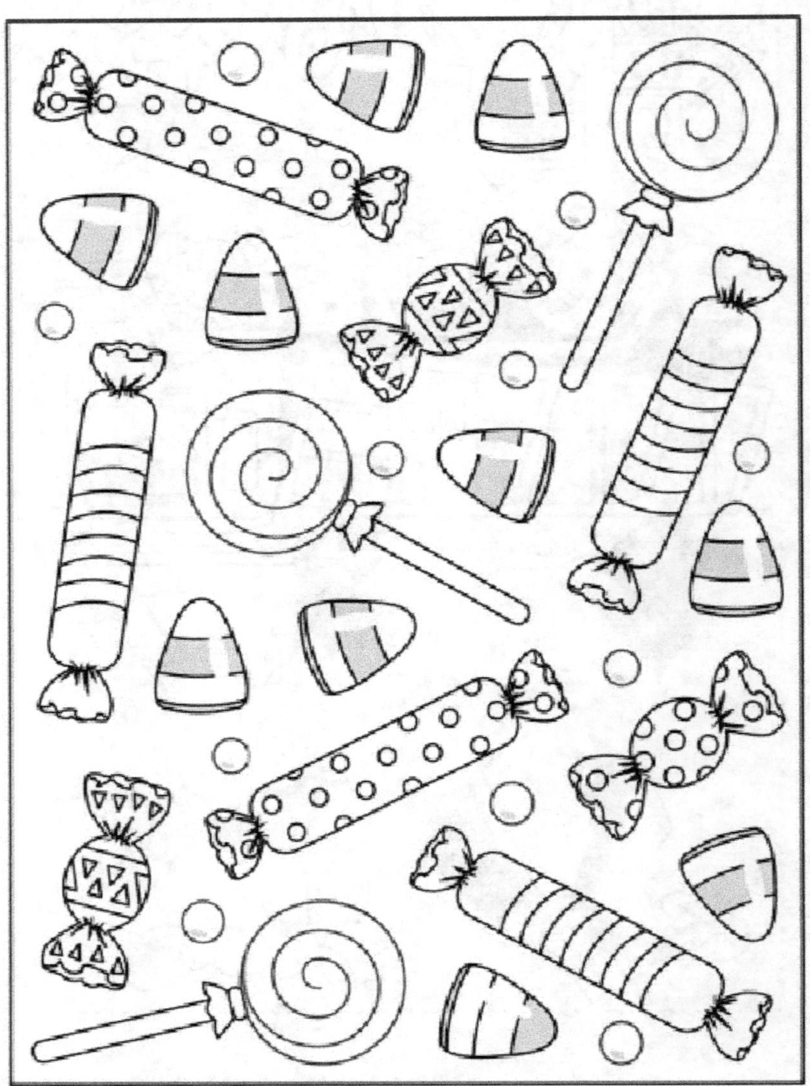

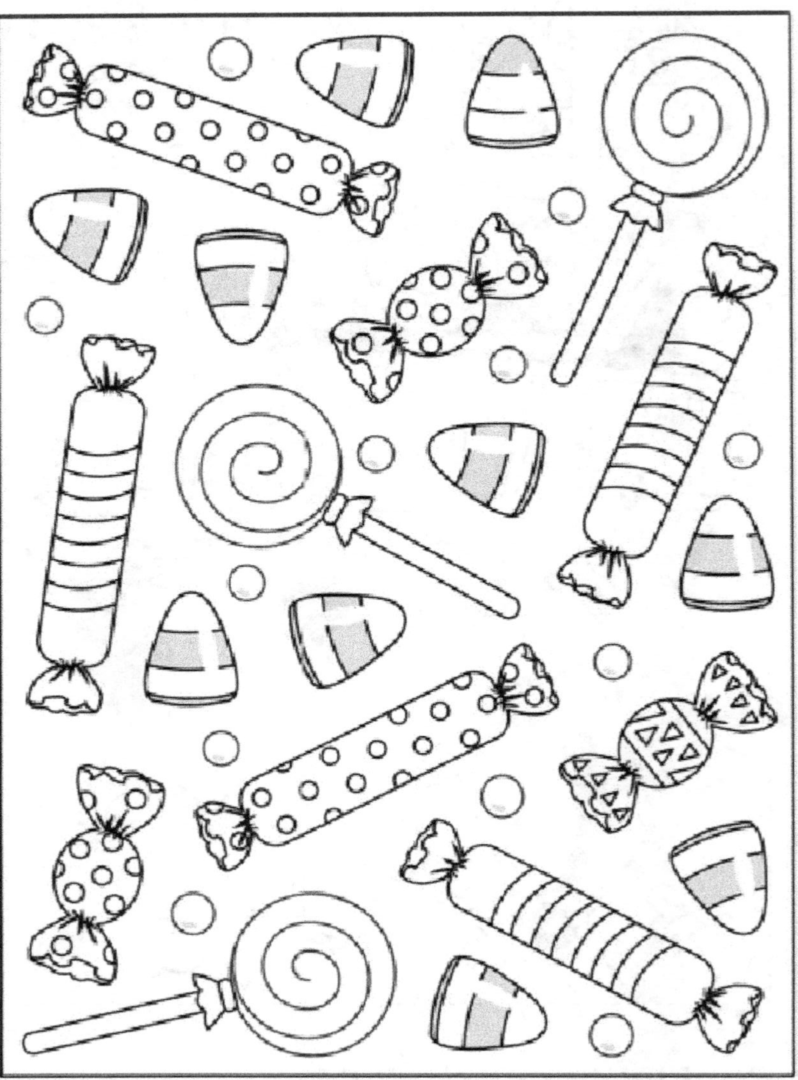

Find the ten differences between the two pictures.

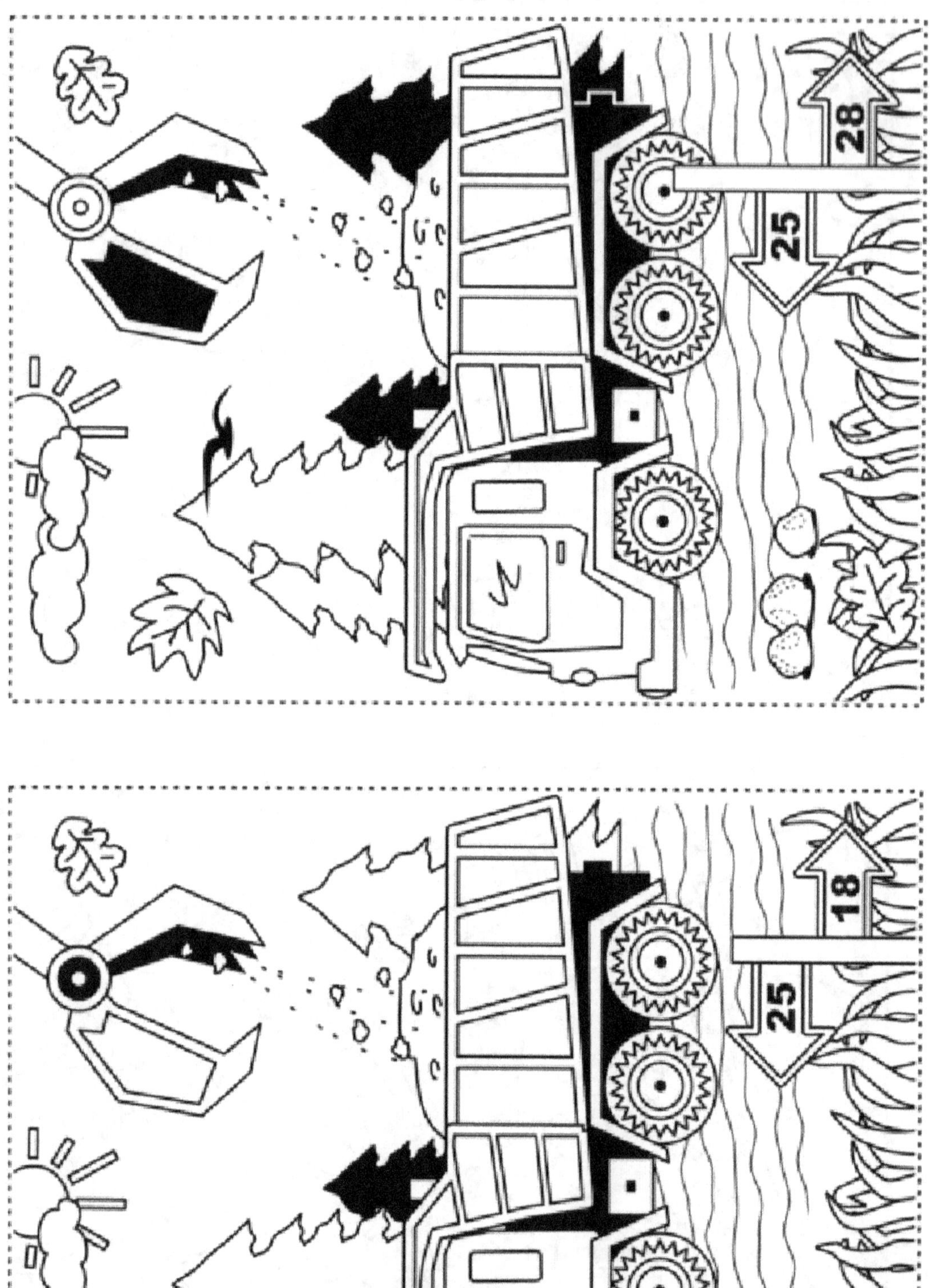

Find 5 differences

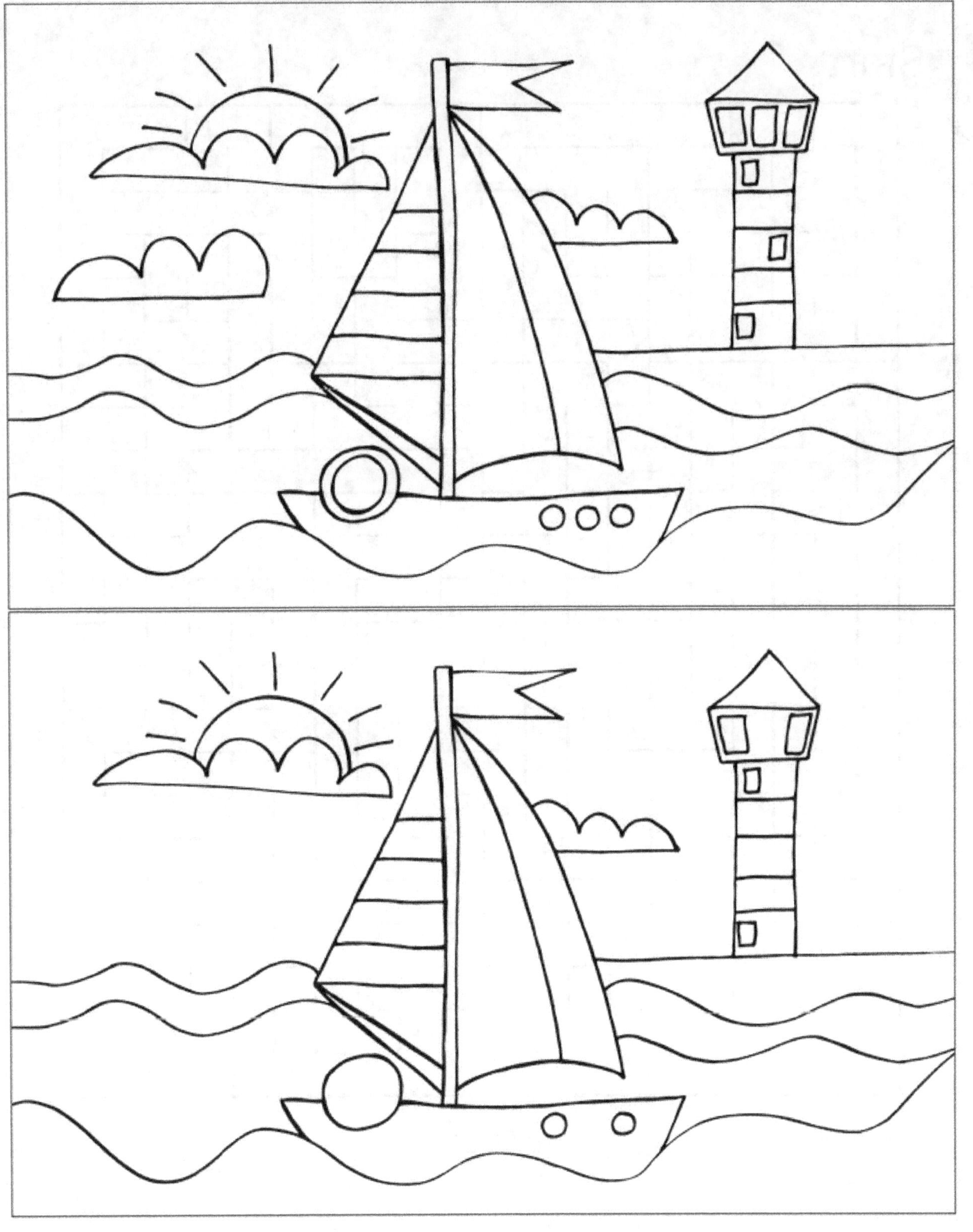

Maze 1

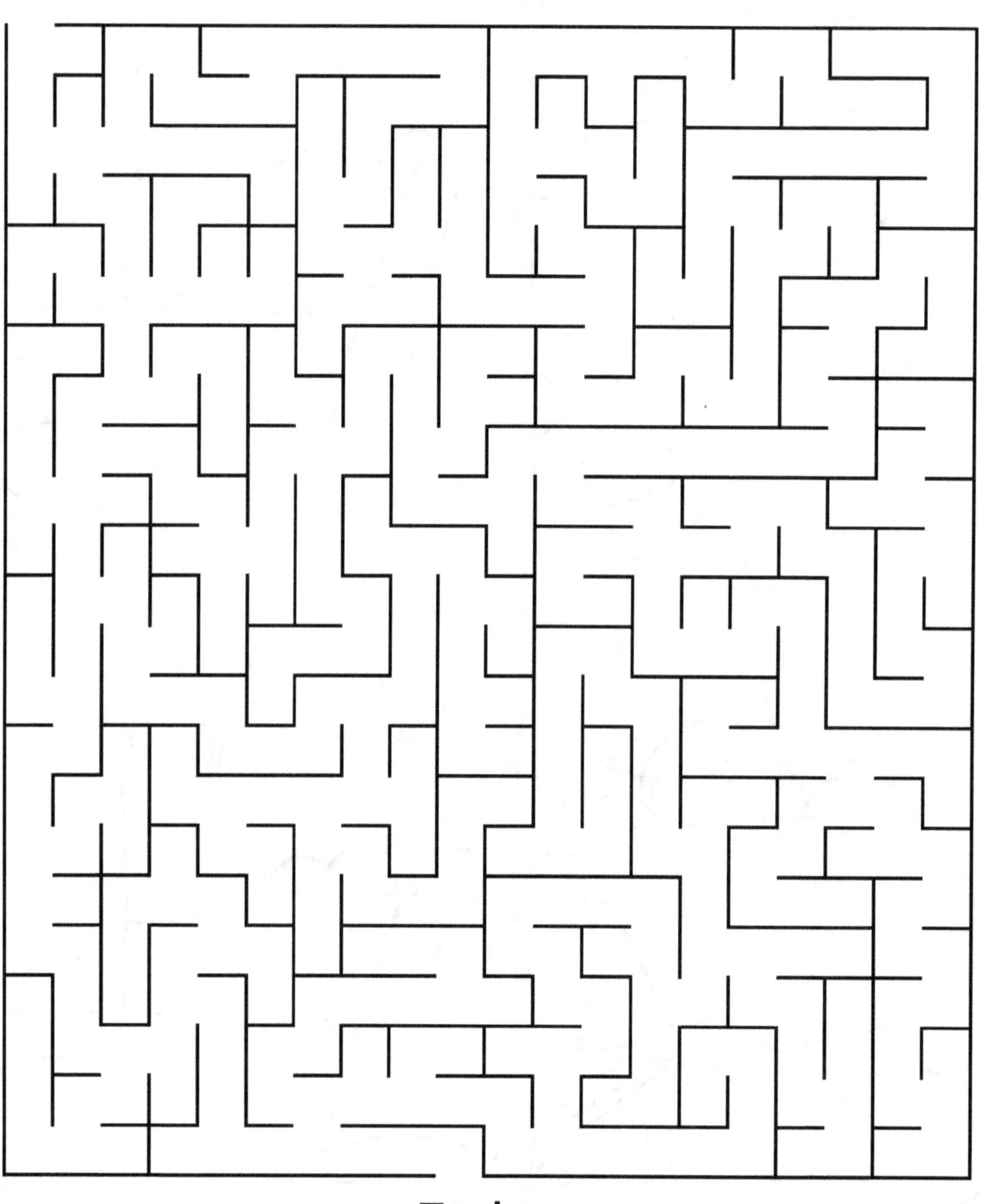

Maze 2

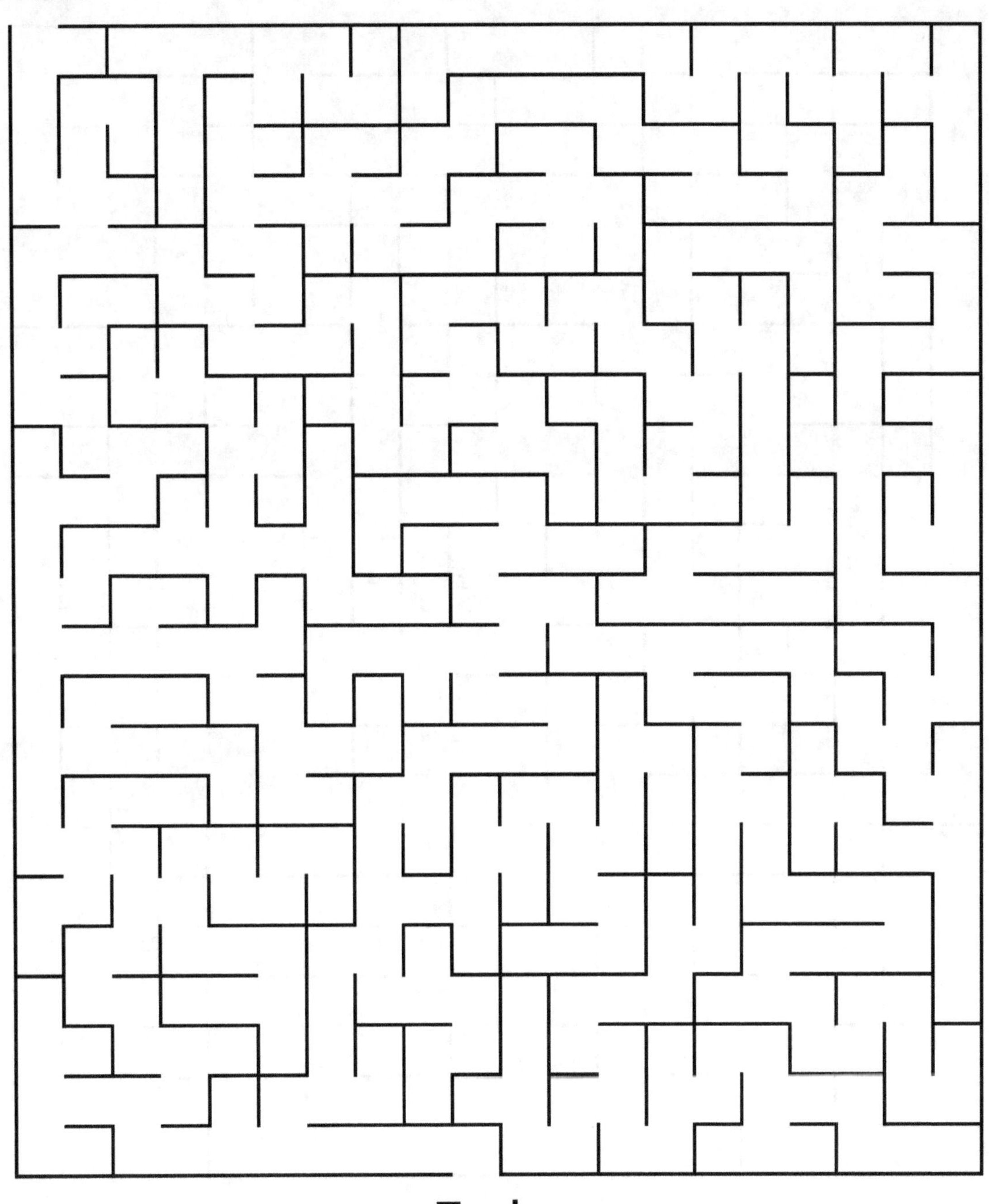

Maze 3

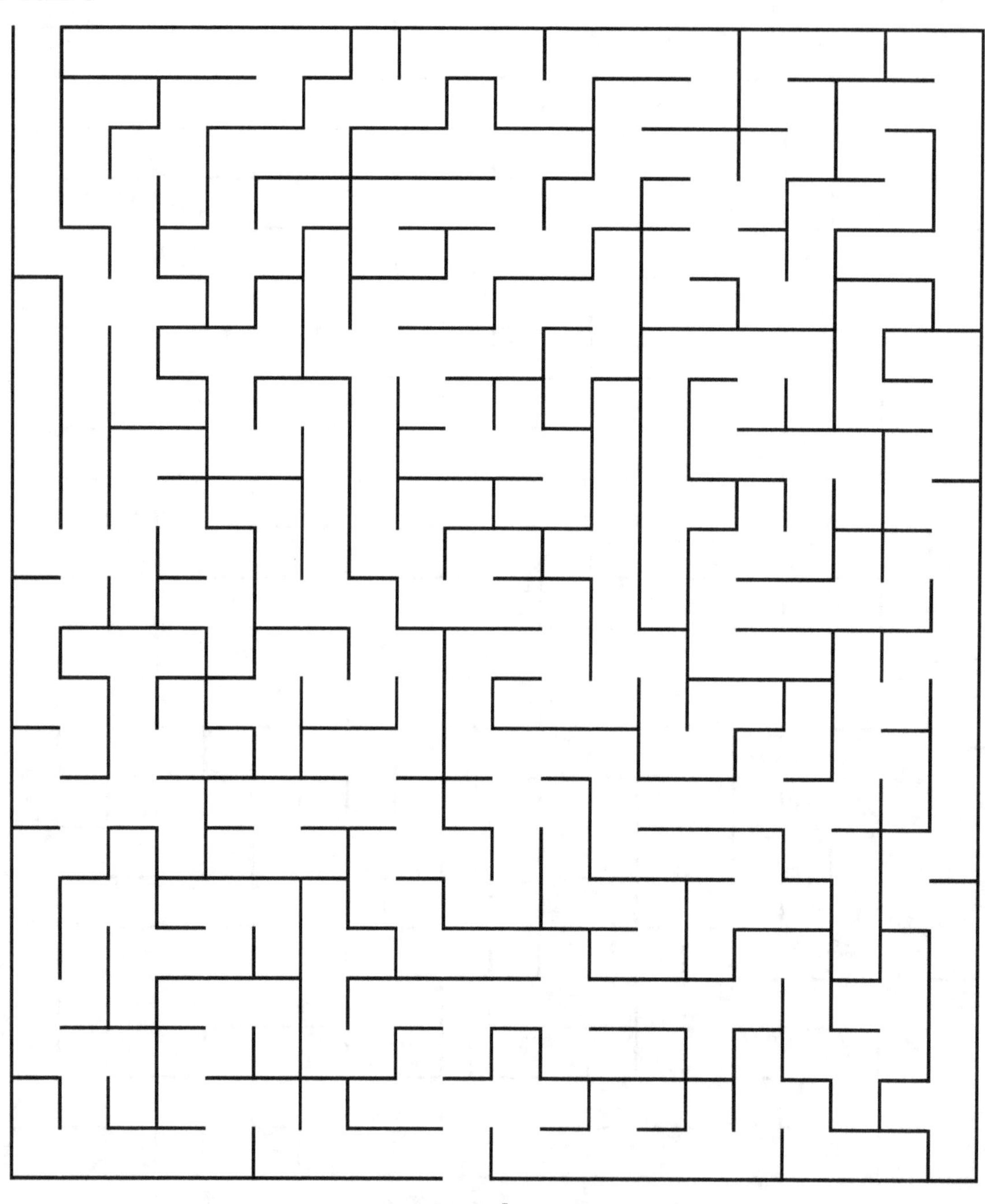

Maze 4

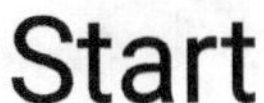

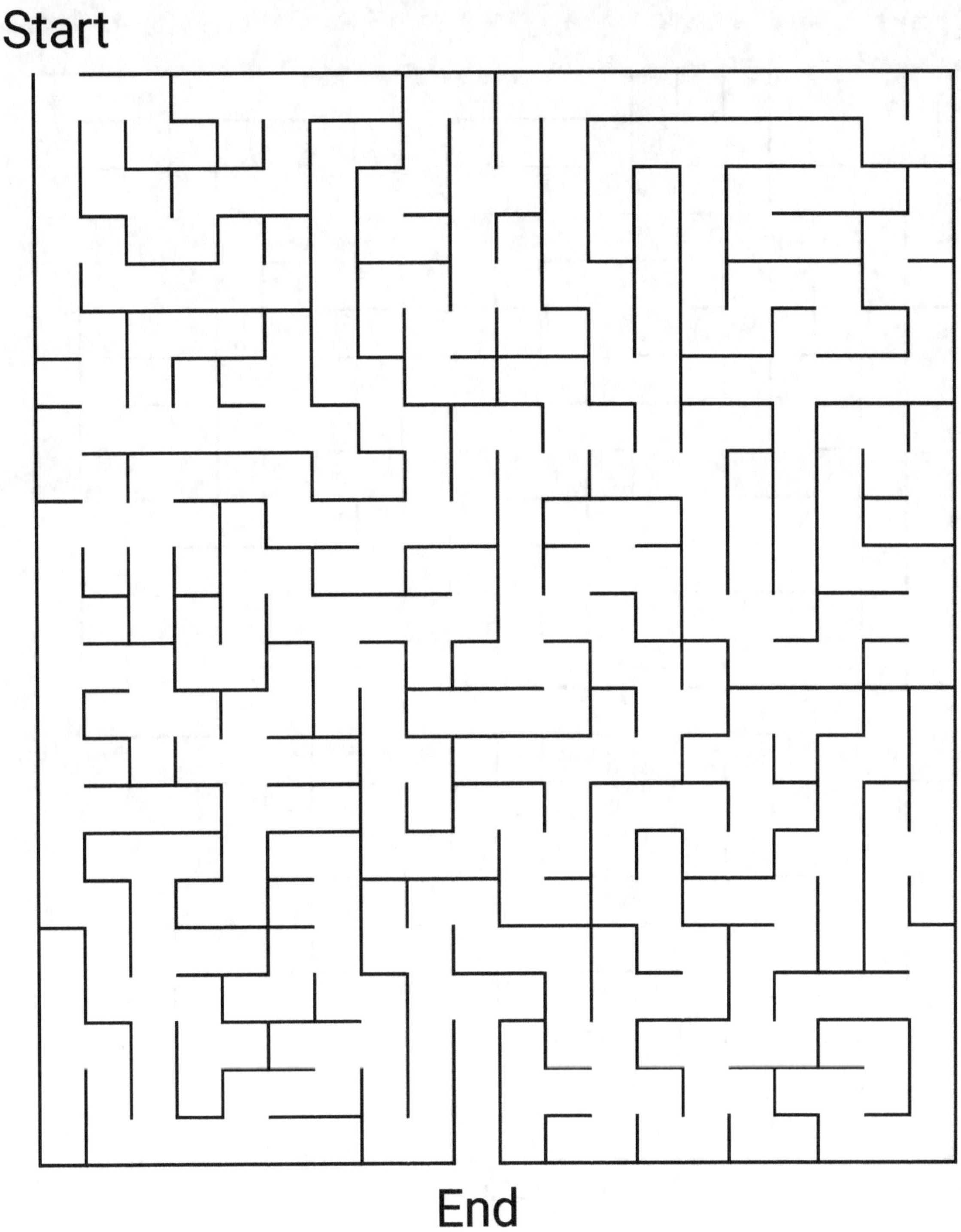

End

Maze 5

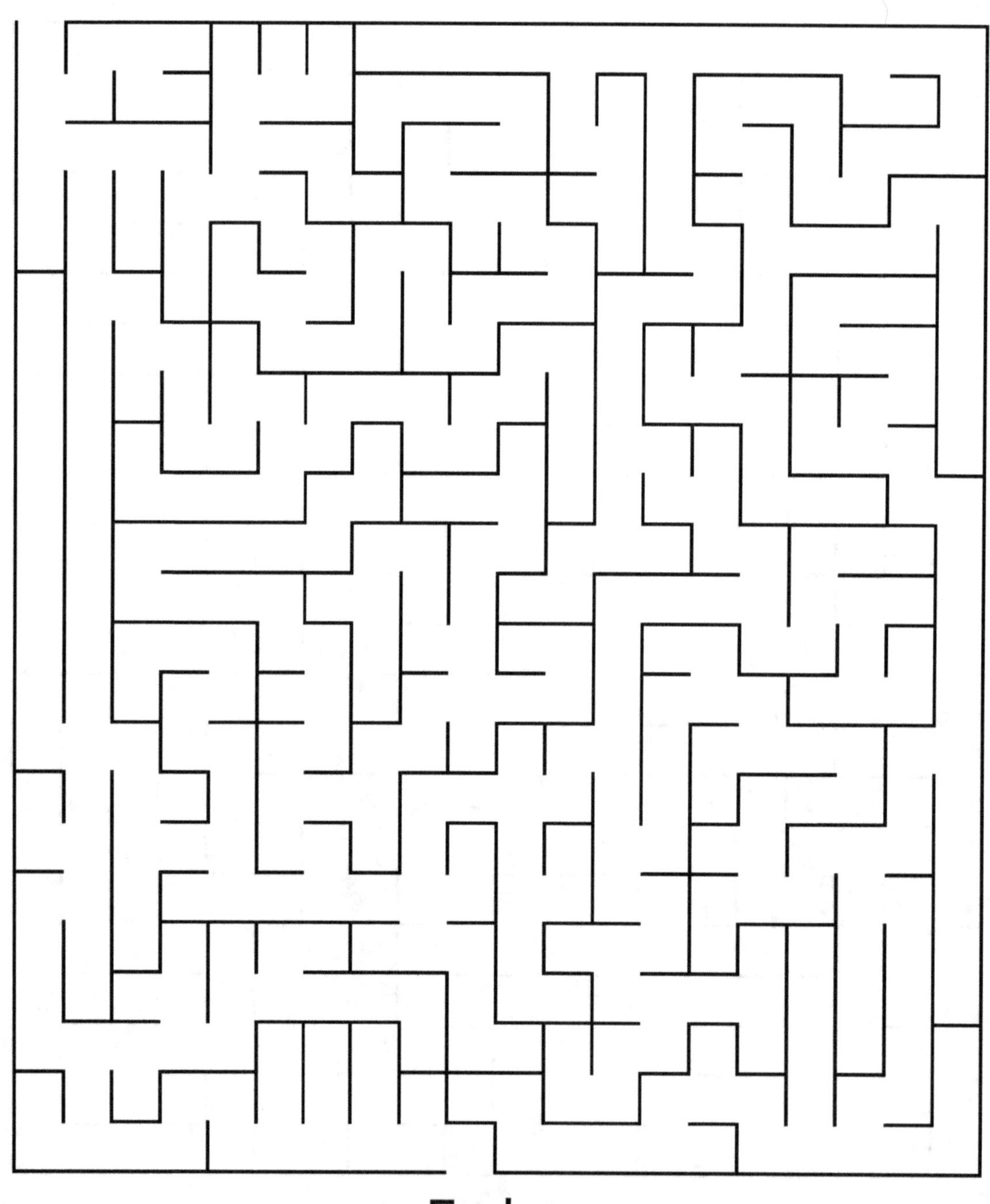

Maze 6

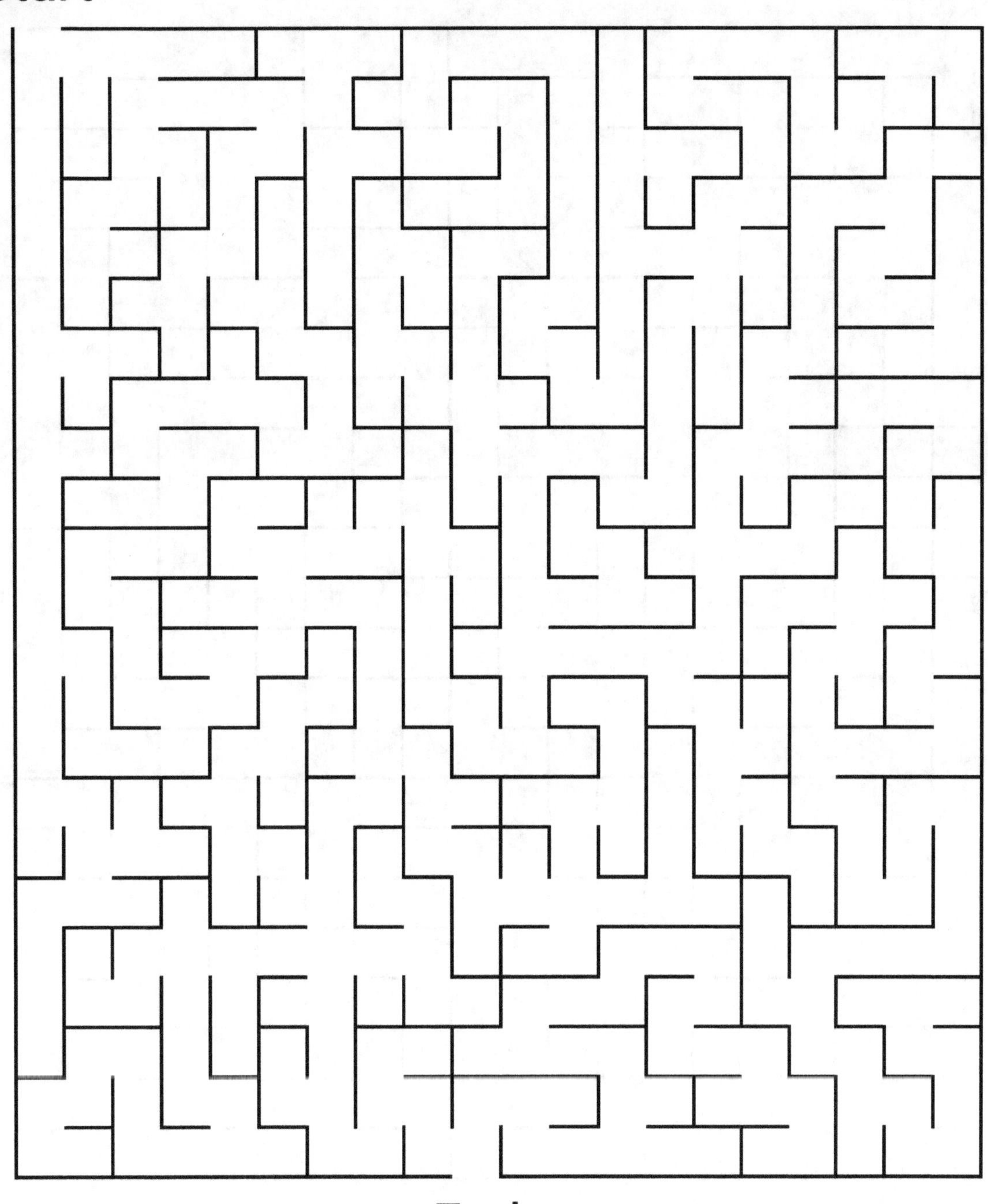

Maze 7

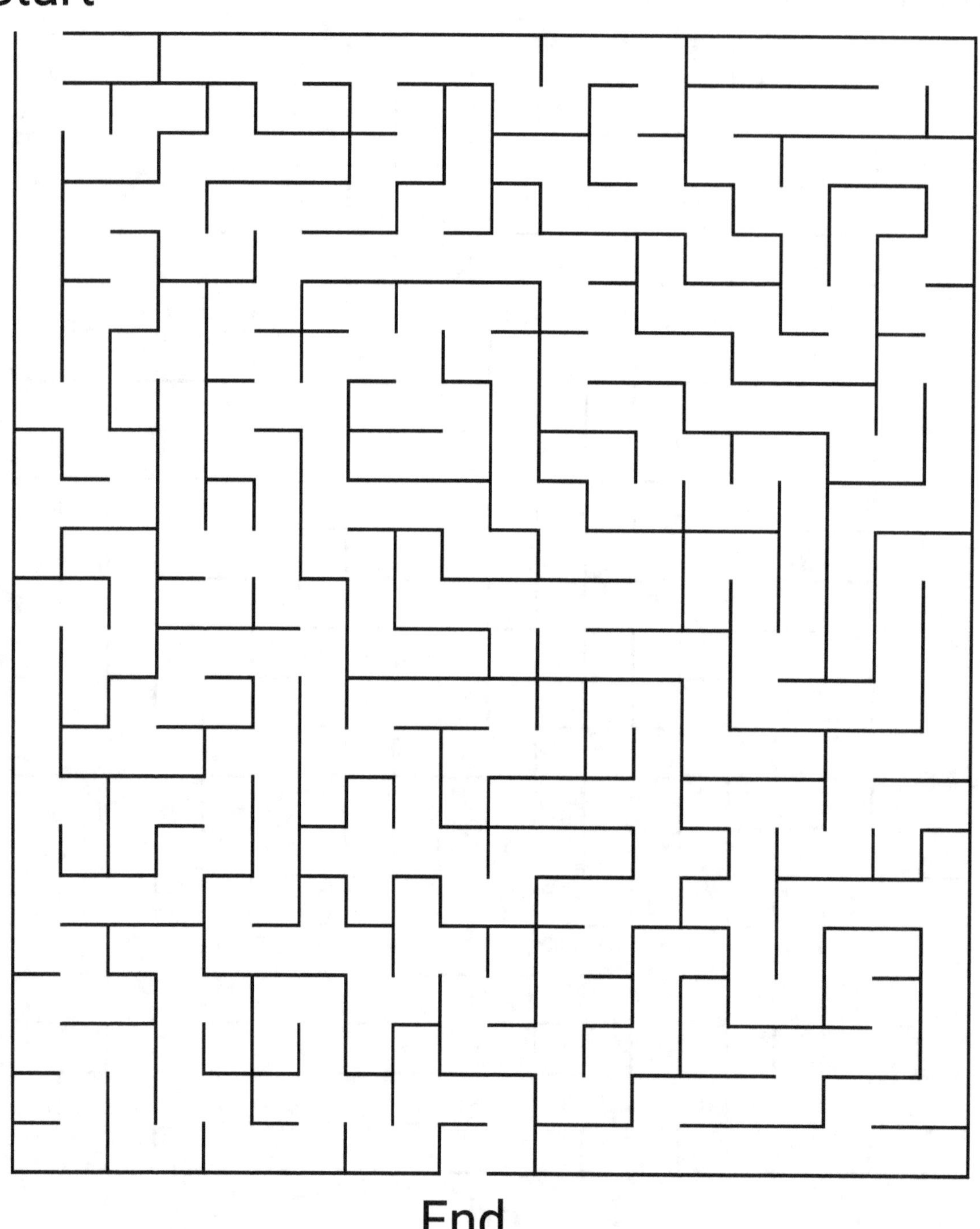

Maze 8

Start

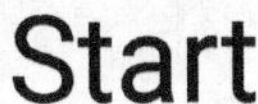

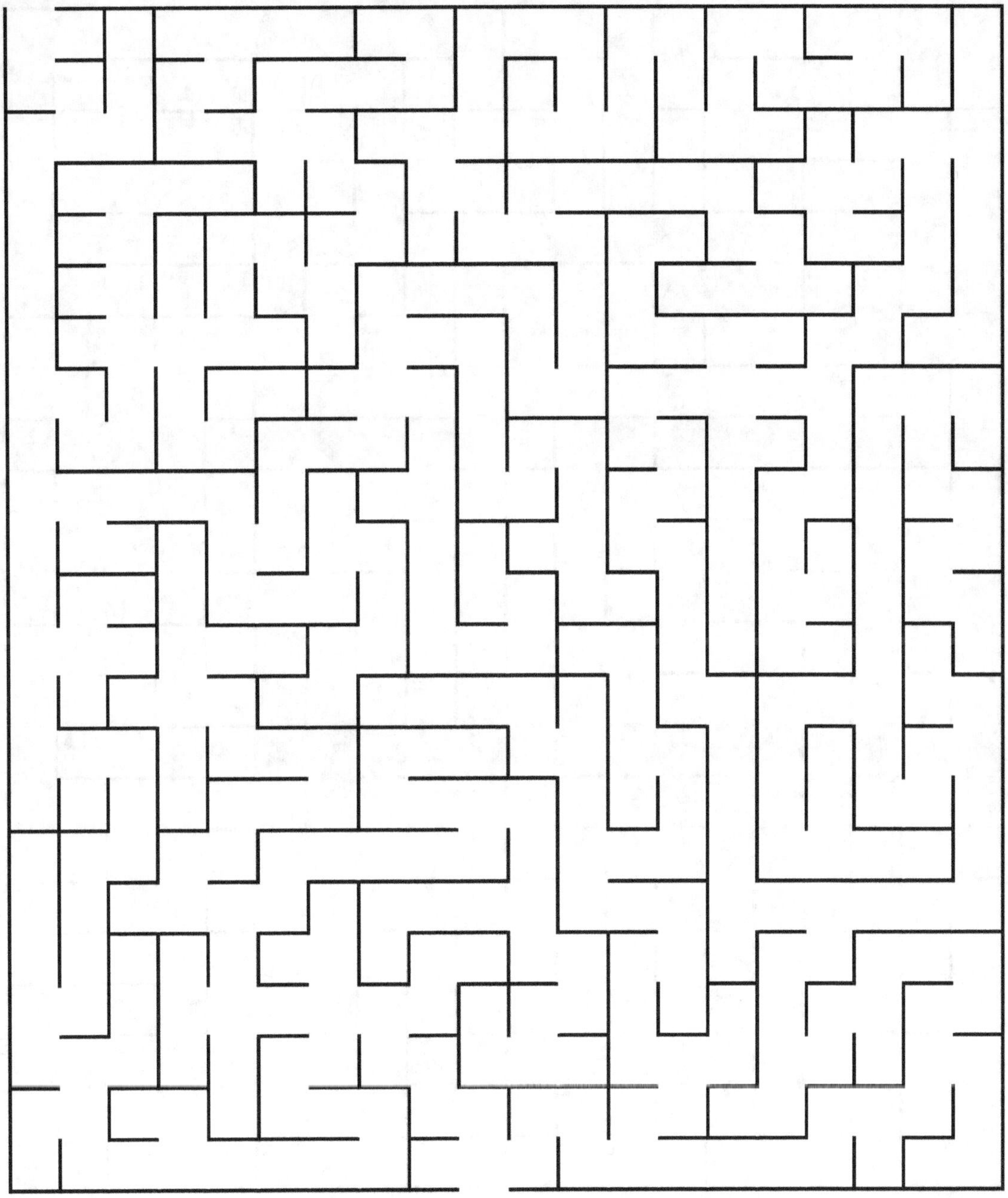

End

Maze 9

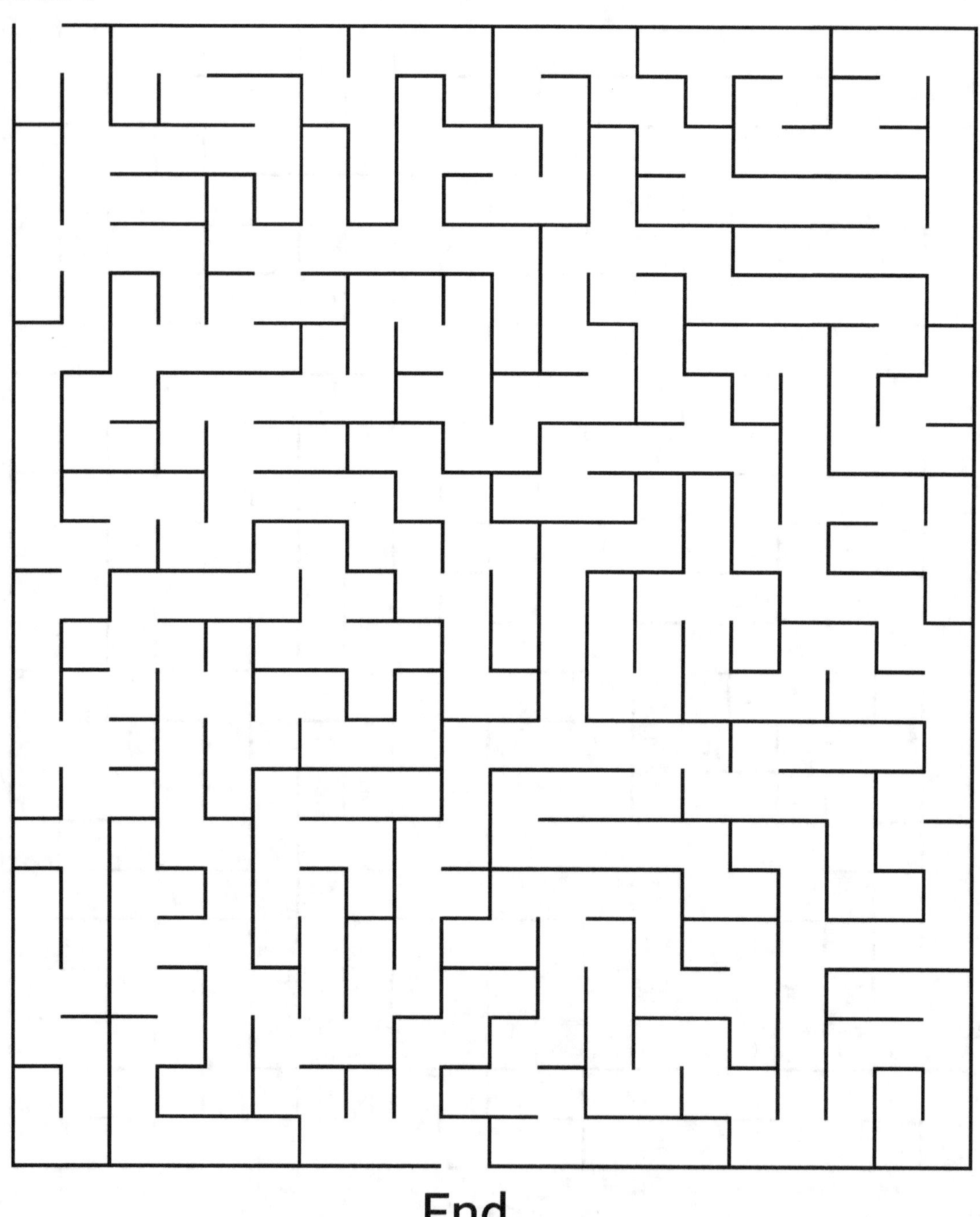

Maze 10

Start

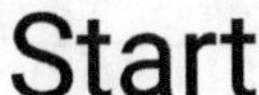

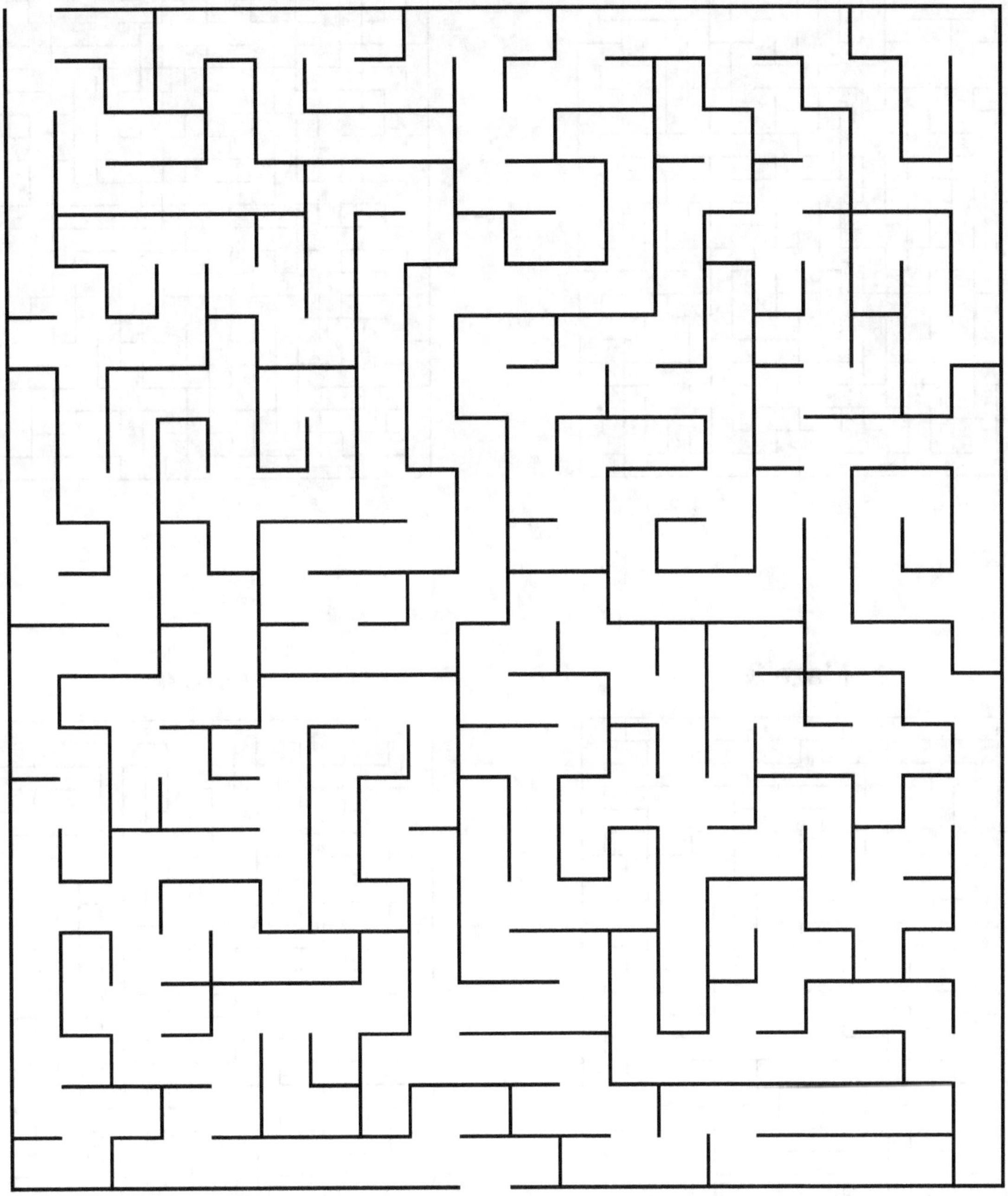

End

Mazes solutions

Maze 1

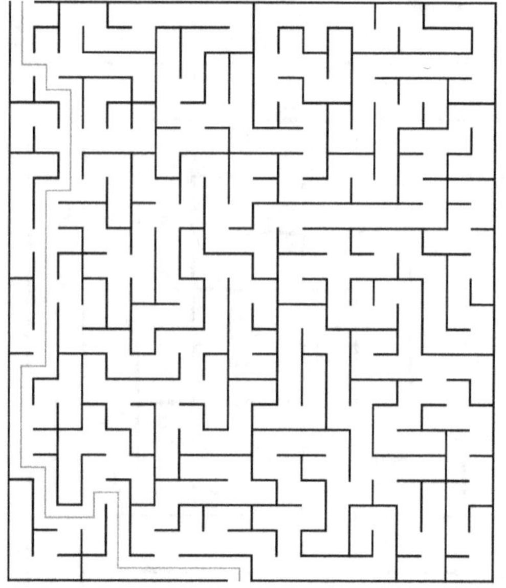

Maze 2

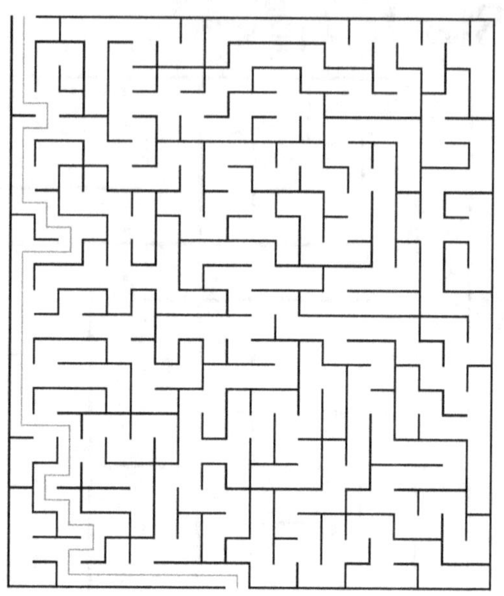

Maze 3

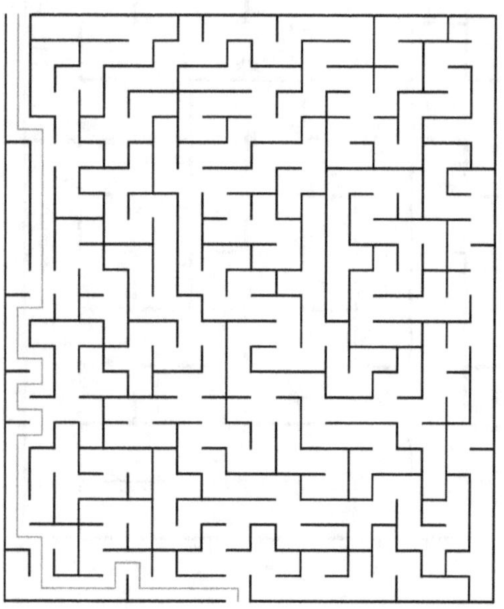

Maze 4

Mazes solutions

Maze 5

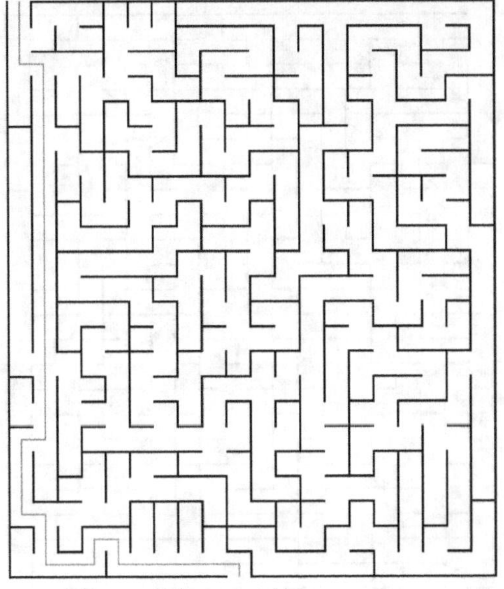

Maze 6

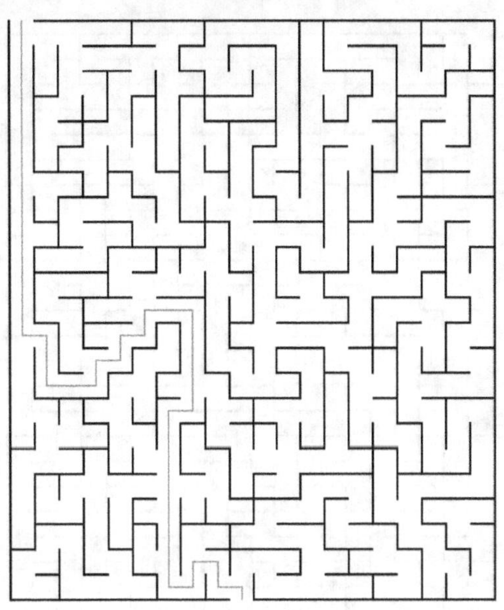

Maze 7

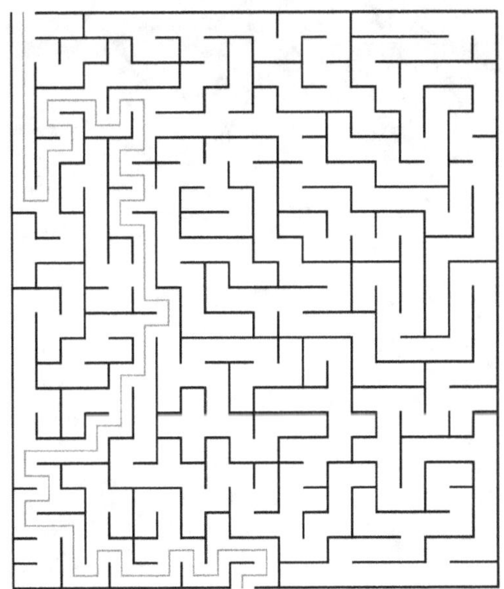

Maze 8

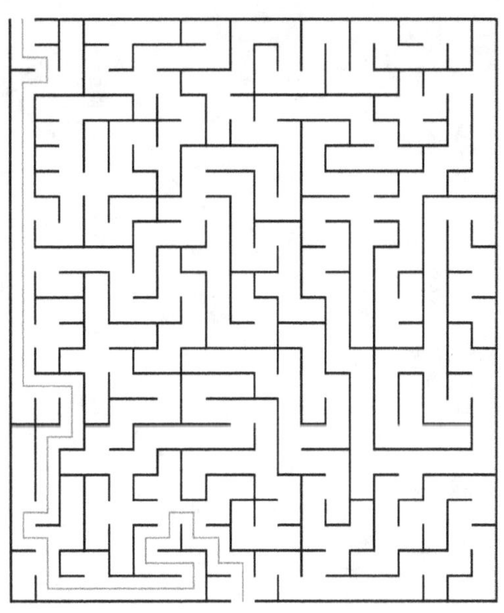

Mazes solutions

Maze 9

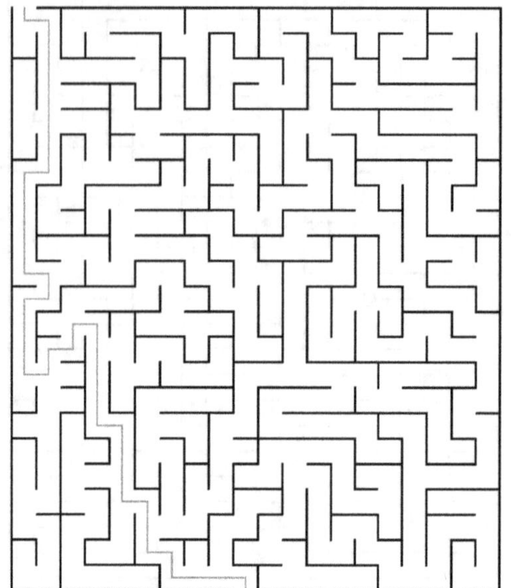

Maze 10

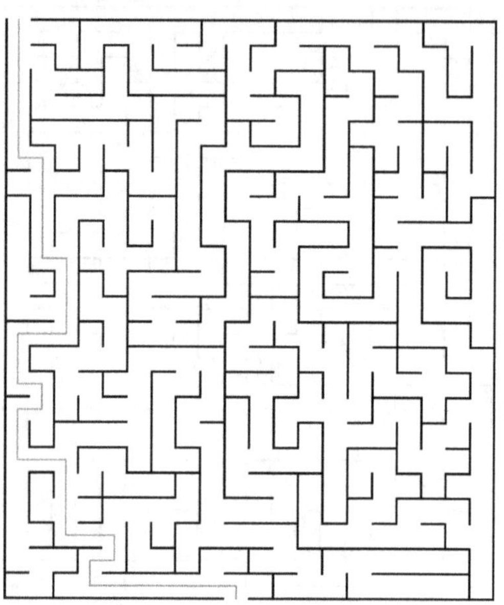

Word Scramble 1

IWHET = _________

DRE = _________

ERGEN = _________

EGRY = _________

EIOVLT = _________

WORNB = _________

NYVA = _________

LNMOE = _________

ABMRE = _________

CCHLOARA = _________

Word List

White	Red	Green
Grey	Violet	Brown
Navy	Lemon	Amber
Charcoal		

Word Scramble 2

ILVEO = _________

BRUY = _______

YIRVO = ________

MDRALEE = ________

BEUL = ________

RUTNBEET = _______

BCKLA = ________

OLEWYL = _______

YKS = _______

LUPREP = _______

Word List

Olive	Ruby	Ivory
Emerald	blue	Brunette
Black	Yellow	Sky
Purple		

Word Scramble 3

NAMGEAT = _______

PNKI = _______

UTESQOIRU = _______

RAGPE = _______

AES = _______

NZREOB = _______

YCNA = _______

ZERAU = _______

TGEANIENR = _______

SPIHPREA = _______

Word List

Magenta   Pink   Turquoise
Grape   Sea   Bronze
Cyan   Azure   Tangerine
Sapphire

Word Scramble 4

EREGN = _________

HAOCM = _______

RENAOG = ________

ELIM = ________

OSINMCR = _______

TADSRUM = _______

CRLAO = ________

TNA = _______

DEERALNV = ________

IGNDOI = _______

Word List

green	Mocha	Orange
Lime	Crimson	Mustard
Coral	Tan	Lavender
Indigo		

Word Scramble 5

ADRK = ______

ERAMC = ______

SLIVER = ______

IMTN = ______

ERRYHC = ______

DOROSOEW = ______

CEOEFF = ______

AHS = ______

OMNROA = ______

MLOSAN = ______

Word List

Dark	Cream	Silver
Mint	Cherry	Rosewood
Coffee	Ash	Maroon
Salmon		

Word Scramble 6

UQAA = _________

CPEHA = _______

RFNFOSA = _________

EALT = _______

BIEEG = _________

FAHUSIC = _________

NDRUUYBG = _________

VMUAE = _________

TRUS = _________

RLPAE = _________

Word List

Aqua	Peach	Saffron
Teal	Beige	Fuchsia
Burgundy	Mauve	Rust
Pearl		

Word Scramble 7

GENART = _______

LCLAI = _______

BURME = _______

LACETJBK = _______

CKHISRWA = _______

LAPERANI = _______

ECBCIYL = _______

KBIE = _______

RAENC = _______

ERRAGCAI = _______

Word List

Garnet	Lilac	Umber
Jet black	Rickshaw	Airplane
Bicycle	Bike	Crane
Carriage		

Word Scramble 8

ANV = _______

RRYFE = _____

ICLTOHREPE = _______

AECPJTK = _______

RROLY = _______

ERTOM = ______

WORAPYE = _______

YTOCSO = ______

TCAROTR = ______

TAE = _______

Word List

Van Ferry Helicopter
Jetpack Lorry Metro
Ropeway Scooty Tractor
Eat

Word Scramble 9

UACLNBAEM = ________

ABTO = ________

USB = ________

ACR = ________

EYLCC = ________

GROAC = ________

UCRTK = ________

ODNLAGOS = ________

OOUAHSBTE = ________

LESIMUNOI = ________

Word List

Ambulance	Boat	Bus
Car	Cycle	Cargo
Truck	Gondolas	Houseboat
Limousine		

Word Scramble 10

MCLYTEORCO = _________

ORWBTOA = _______

HIPS = ______

OOERTCS = ________

RTAIN = _______

RNIDK = ________

AEGEL = ________

CCEAKOP = ________

INOEGP = _______

ARKEEAPT = _______

Word List

Motorcycle

Scooter

Eagle

Parakeet

Rowboat

Train

Peacock

Ship

Drink

Pigeon

Word scramble solutions

Word Scramble 1

IWHET = WHITE

DRE = RED

ERGEN = GREEN

EGRY = GREY

EIOVLT = VIOLET

WORNB = BROWN

NYVA = NAVY

LNMOE = LEMON

ABMRE = AMBER

CCHLOARA = CHARCOAL

Word Scramble 2

ILVEO = OLIVE

BRUY = RUBY

YIRVO = IVORY

MDRALEE = EMERALD

BEUL = BLUE

RUTNBEET = BRUNETTE

BCKLA = BLACK

OLEWYL = YELLOW

YKS = SKY

LUPREP = PURPLE

Word Scramble 3

NAMGEAT = MAGENTA

PNKI = PINK

UTESQOIRU = TURQUOISE

RAGPE = GRAPE

AES = SEA

NZREOB = BRONZE

YCNA = CYAN

ZERAU = AZURE

TGEANIENR = TANGERINE

SPIHPREA = SAPPHIRE

Word Scramble 4

EREGN = GREEN

HAOCM = MOCHA

RENAOG = ORANGE

ELIM = LIME

OSINMCR = CRIMSON

TADSRUM = MUSTARD

CRLAO = CORAL

TNA = TAN

DEERALNV = LAVENDER

IGNDOI = INDIGO

Word scramble solutions

Word Scramble 5

ADRK = DARK

ERAMC = CREAM

SLIVER = SILVER

IMTN = MINT

ERRYHC = CHERRY

DOROSOEW = ROSEWOOD

CEOEFF = COFFEE

AHS = ASH

OMNROA = MAROON

MLOSAN = SALMON

Word Scramble 6

UQAA = AQUA

CPEHA = PEACH

RFNFOSA = SAFFRON

EALT = TEAL

BIEEG = BEIGE

FAHUSIC = FUCHSIA

NDRUUYBG = BURGUNDY

VMUAE = MAUVE

TRUS = RUST

RLPAE = PEARL

Word Scramble 7

GENART = GARNET

LCLAI = LILAC

BURME = UMBER

LACETJBK = JET BLACK

CKHISRWA = RICKSHAW

LAPERANI = AIRPLANE

ECBCIYL = BICYCLE

KBIE = BIKE

RAENC = CRANE

ERRAGCAI = CARRIAGE

Word Scramble 8

ANV = VAN

RRYFE = FERRY

ICLTOHREPE = HELICOPTER

AECPJTK = JETPACK

RROLY = LORRY

ERTOM = METRO

WORAPYE = ROPEWAY

YTOCSO = SCOOTY

TCAROTR = TRACTOR

TAE = EAT

Word scramble solutions

Word Scramble 9

UACLNBAEM = AMBULANCE

ABTO = BOAT

USB = BUS

ACR = CAR

EYLCC = CYCLE

GROAC = CARGO

UCRTK = TRUCK

ODNLAGOS = GONDOLAS

OOUAHSBTE = HOUSEBOAT

LESIMUNOI = LIMOUSINE

Word Scramble 10

MCLYTEORCO = MOTORCYCLE

ORWBTOA = ROWBOAT

HIPS = SHIP

OOERTCS = SCOOTER

RTAIN = TRAIN

RNIDK = DRINK

AEGEL = EAGLE

CCEAKOP = PEACOCK

INOEGP = PIGEON

ARKEEAPT = PARAKEET

Telling Time

Write the time inside each clock below

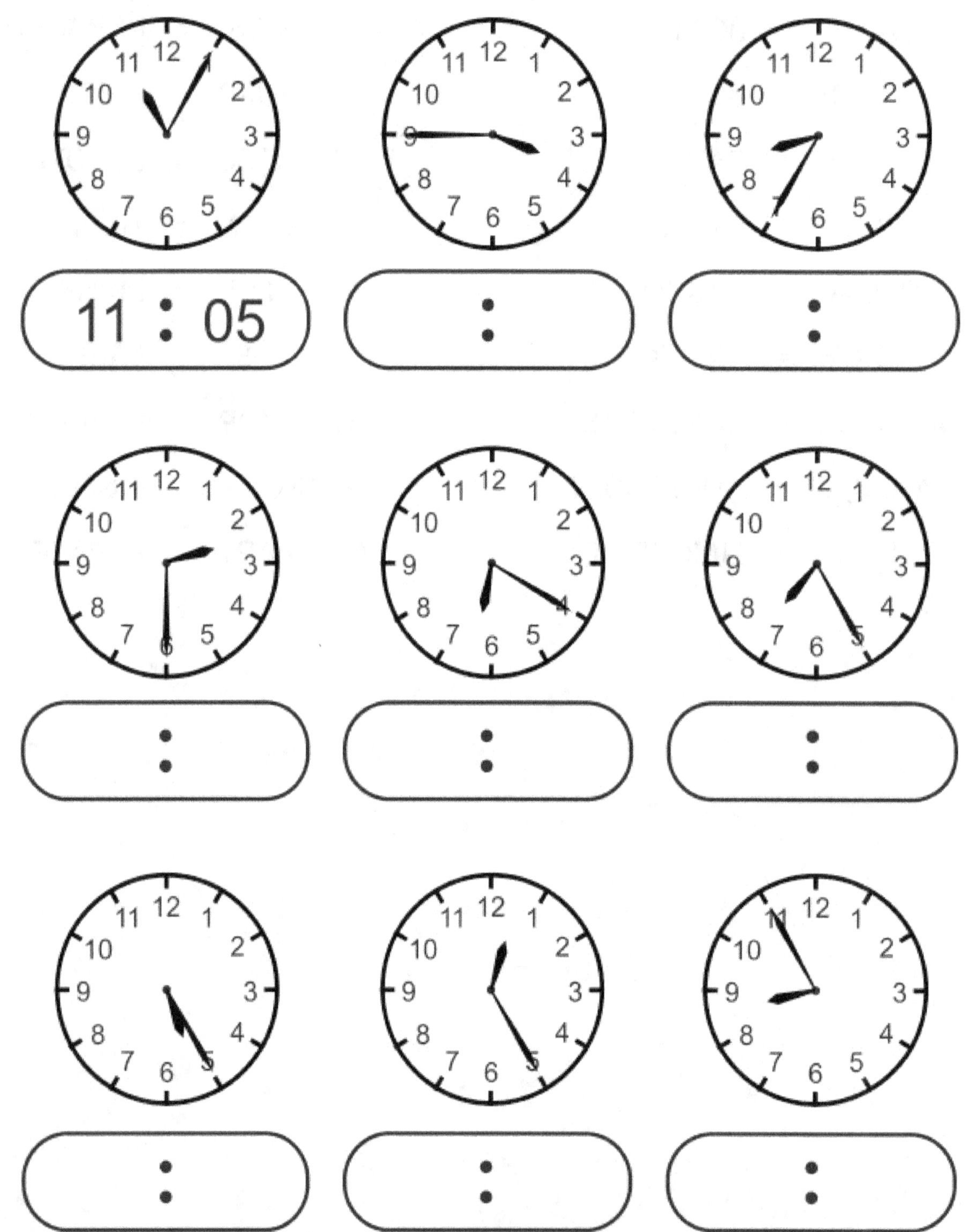

Telling Time

Write the time inside each clock below

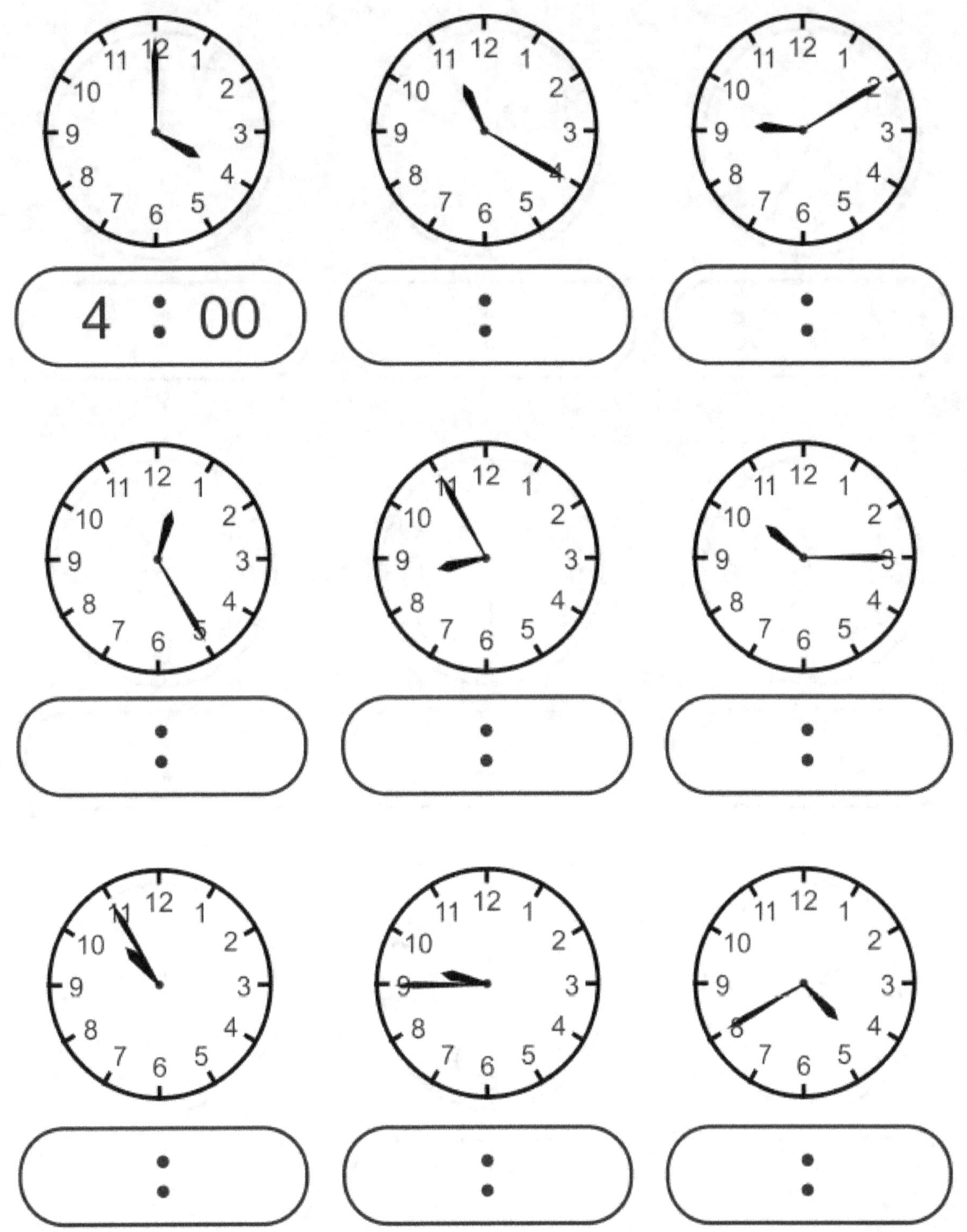

Telling Time

Write the time inside each clock below

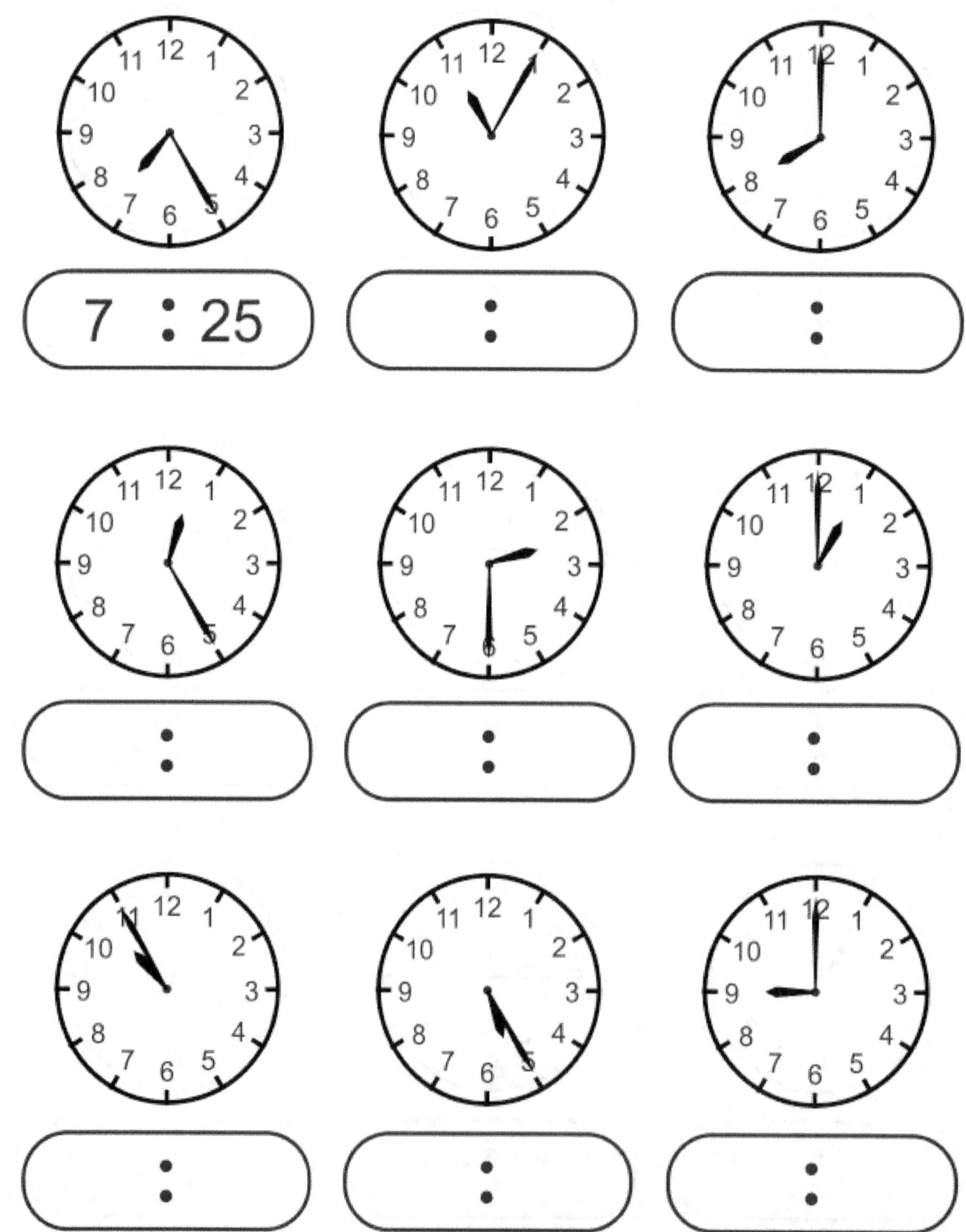

7 : 25

Telling Time

Write the time inside each clock below

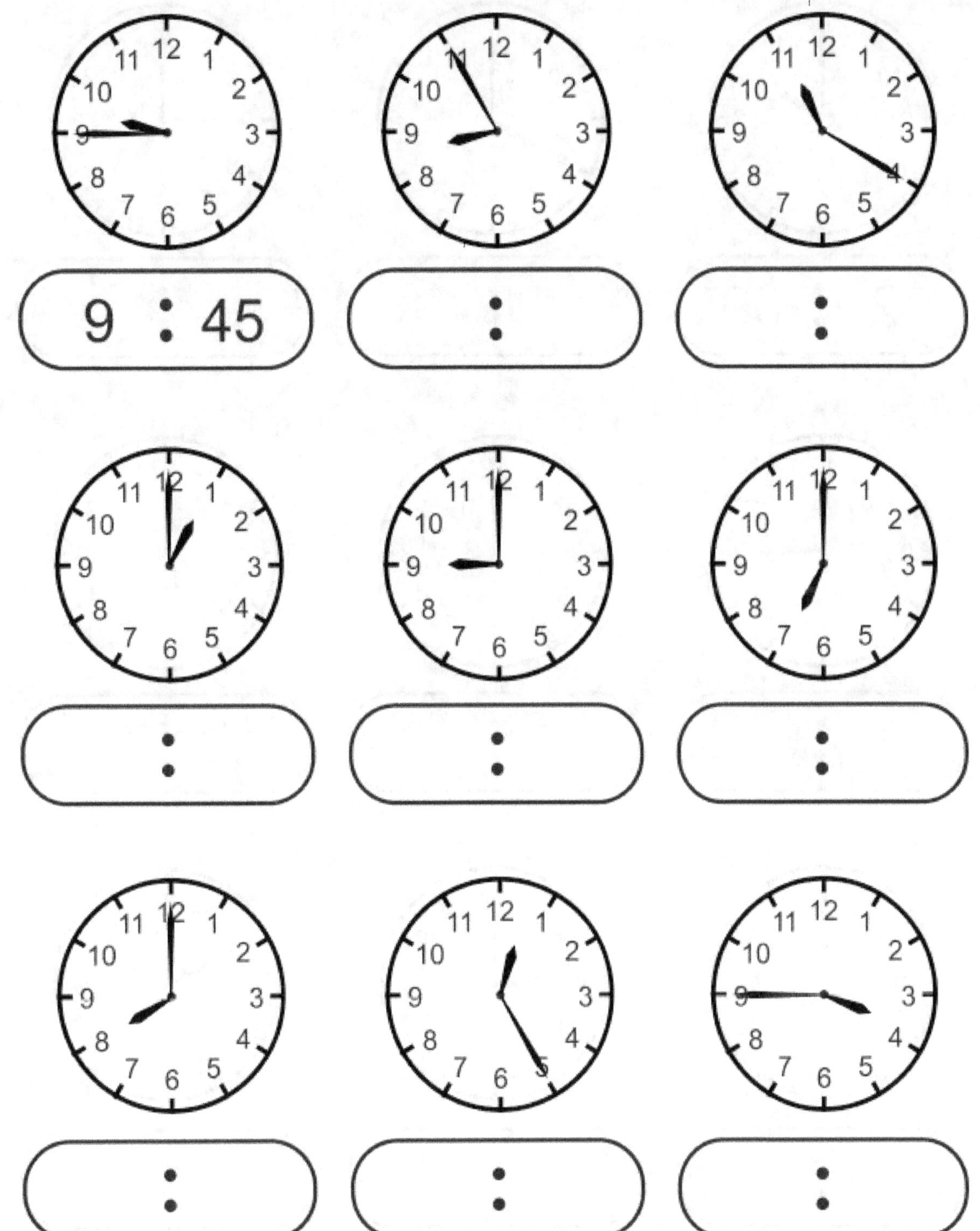

9 : 45

Telling Time

Write the time inside each clock below

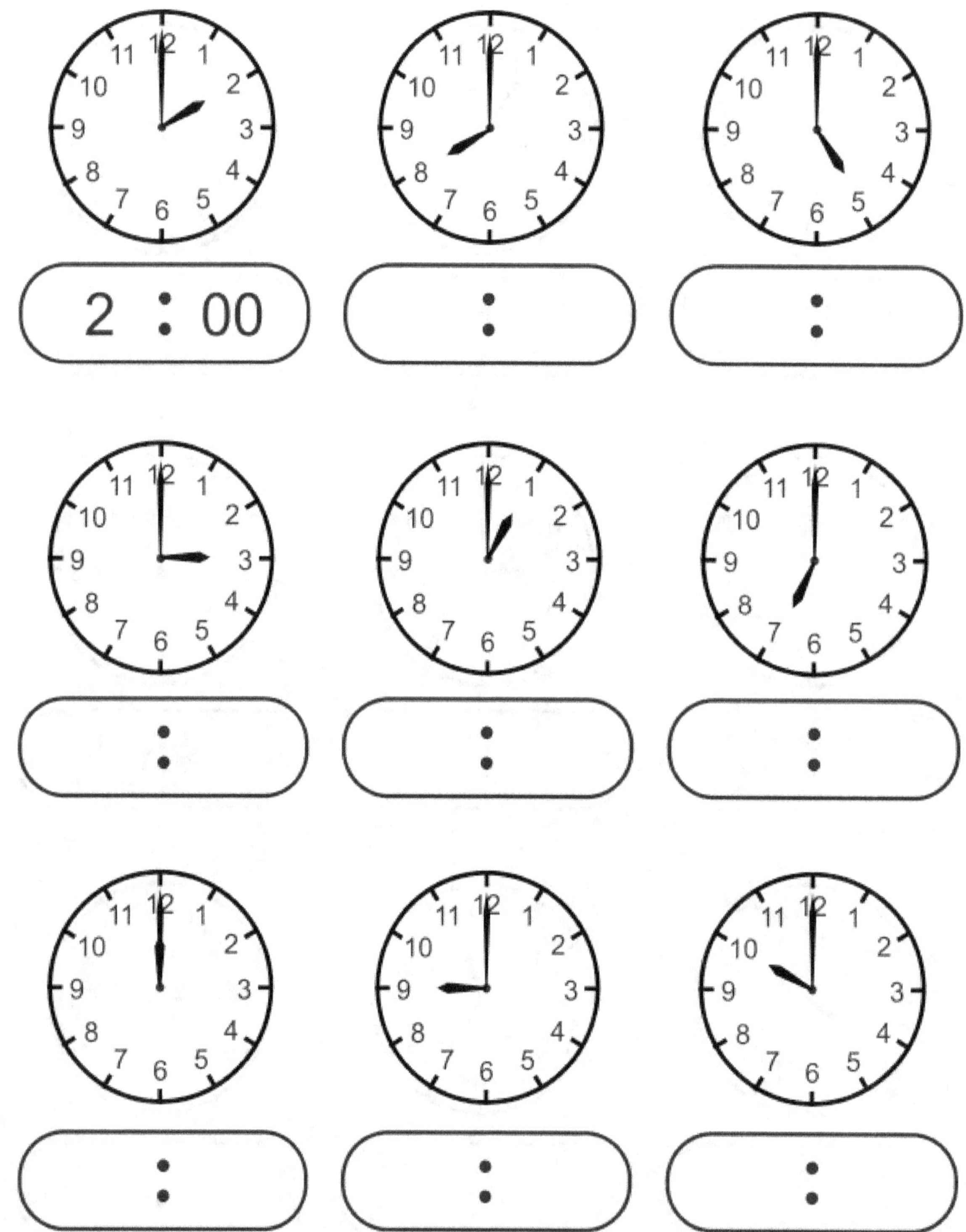

Telling Time

Draw a line to connect the matching times.

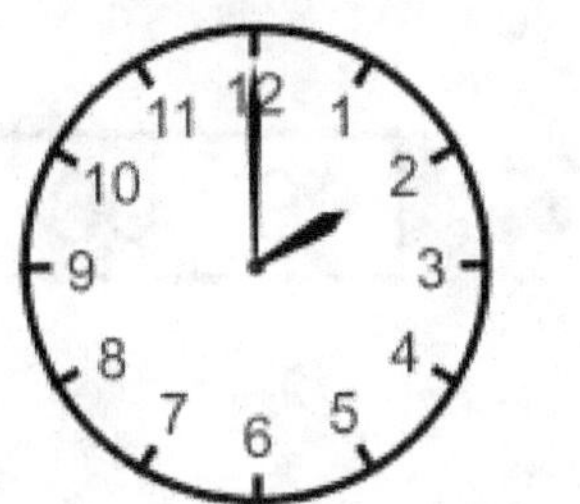 •   • | 8 : 00 |

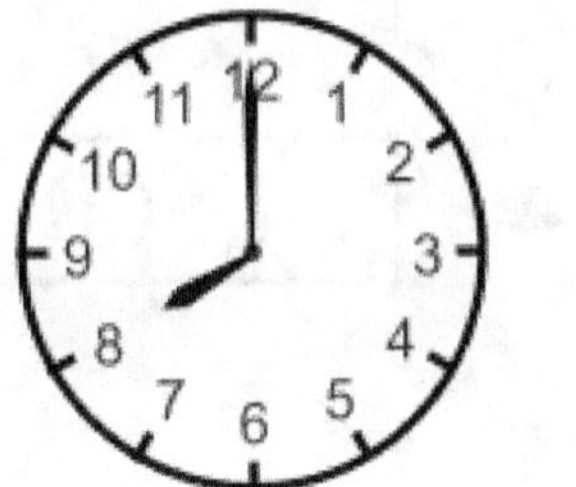 •   • | 2 : 00 |

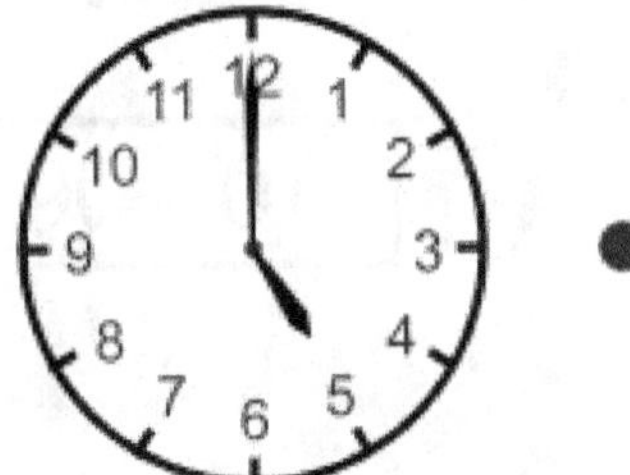 •   • | 1 : 00 |

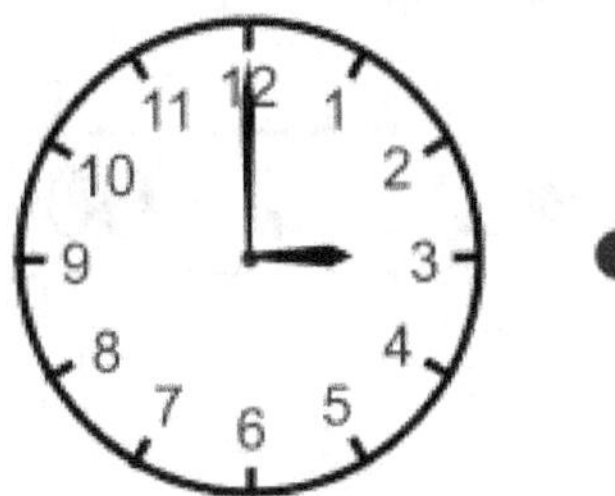 •   • | 5 : 00 |

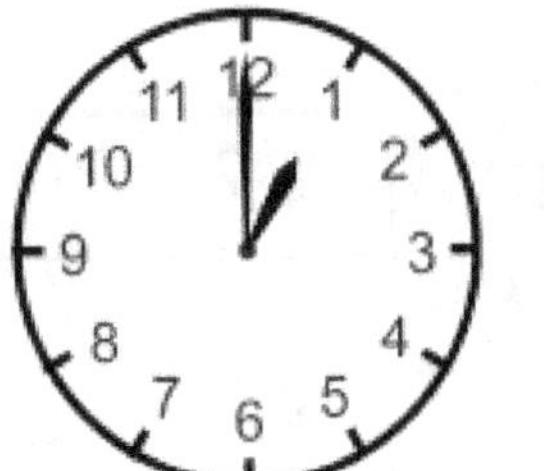 •   • | 3 : 00 |

Telling Time

Draw a line to connect the matching times.

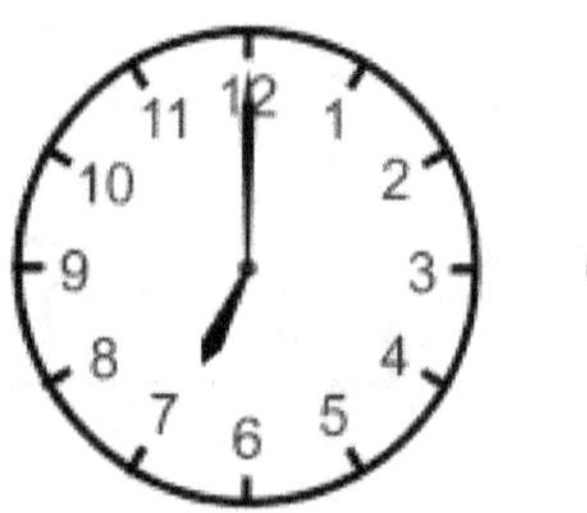

•   •   9 : 00

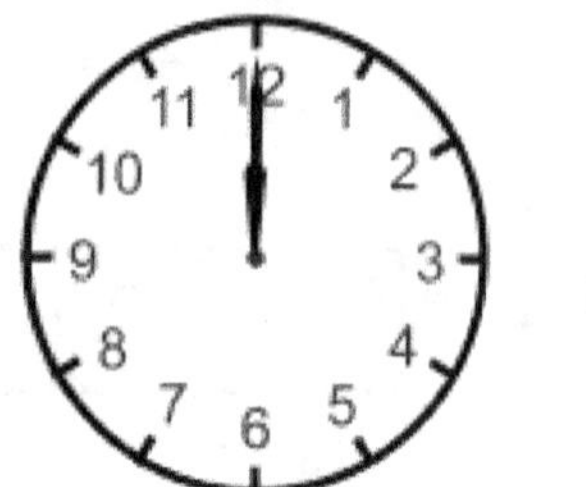

•   •   4 : 00

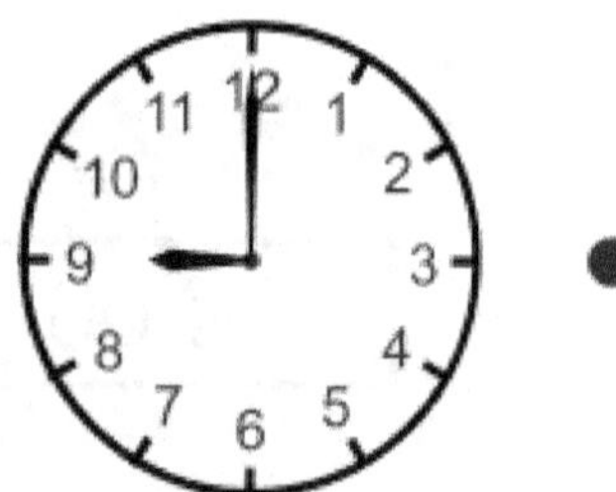

•   •   10 : 00

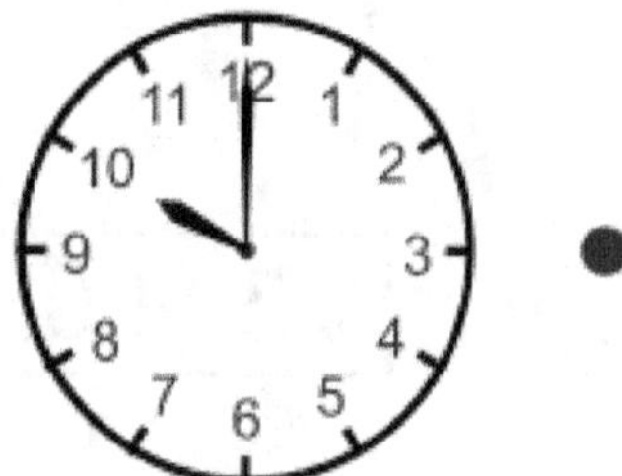

•   •   7 : 00

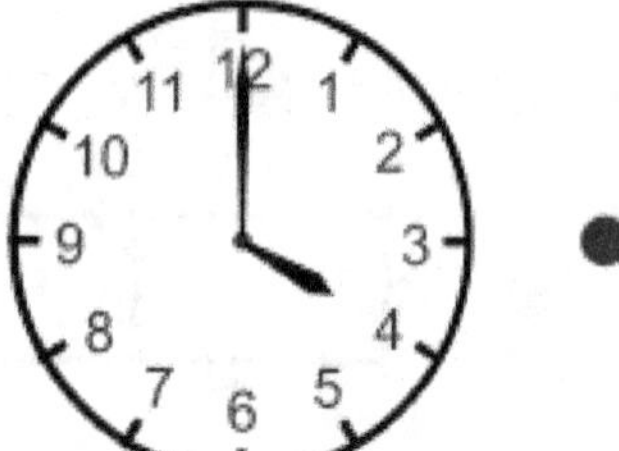

•   •   12 : 00

Sudoku 1

		6	3		
2	1	3			
6				3	
	4	5			
	6		5	4	3
5	3	4		2	6

Sudoku 2

6			1	5	
1	2			4	
3	6	2			5
	5	1	2	6	
5	4				
		6	5		

Sudoku 3

			5	1	2
	2				
2			4		3
	4	6		5	
6	1			4	5
5			1		6

Sudoku 4

	1				4
		4		3	1
6	4				5
		1			
4	6		1	2	3
1	2	3			6

Sudoku 5

<table>
<tr><td>6</td><td></td><td></td><td></td><td>4</td><td>5</td></tr>
<tr><td>4</td><td></td><td></td><td>2</td><td>3</td><td>6</td></tr>
<tr><td></td><td></td><td>3</td><td></td><td></td><td>2</td></tr>
<tr><td>5</td><td></td><td>6</td><td>3</td><td></td><td></td></tr>
<tr><td></td><td></td><td></td><td>5</td><td></td><td>1</td></tr>
<tr><td>2</td><td>5</td><td></td><td>4</td><td>6</td><td></td></tr>
</table>

Sudoku 6

Sudoku 7

	6	4			
3			4	6	
5					
				4	
1	5		3	2	
4	2			1	5

Sudoku 8

	1			2	
	2			6	4
4	3		2	5	
		2	5		
6		3		4	

Sudoku 9

	1	3		5	
	4				3
				4	6
	5	6	2	3	
	2	5		1	
	6				

Sudoku 10

Sudoku 11

	1				
4		2	1	3	
2	3		5		
		5		4	
3				2	
		6	3		

Sudoku 12

Sudoku 13

Sudoku 14

Sudoku 15

				2	
		3			4
	2	4		5	
5		2	6		1
	6		2	3	5

Sudoku solutions

Sudoku 1

4	5	6	3	1	2
2	1	3	6	5	4
6	2	1	4	3	5
3	4	5	2	6	1
1	6	2	5	4	3
5	3	4	1	2	6

Sudoku 2

6	3	4	1	5	2
1	2	5	3	4	6
3	6	2	4	1	5
4	5	1	2	6	3
5	4	3	6	2	1
2	1	6	5	3	4

Sudoku 3

4	6	3	5	1	2
1	2	5	6	3	4
2	5	1	4	6	3
3	4	6	2	5	1
6	1	2	3	4	5
5	3	4	1	2	6

Sudoku 4

3	1	6	2	5	4
2	5	4	6	3	1
6	4	2	3	1	5
5	3	1	4	6	2
4	6	5	1	2	3
1	2	3	5	4	6

Sudoku solutions

Sudoku 5

6	3	2	1	4	5
4	1	5	2	3	6
1	4	3	6	5	2
5	2	6	3	1	4
3	6	4	5	2	1
2	5	1	4	6	3

Sudoku 6

2	3	4	6	1	5
6	5	1	3	2	4
3	2	5	1	4	6
4	1	6	2	5	3
1	4	3	5	6	2
5	6	2	4	3	1

Sudoku 7

2	6	4	1	5	3
3	1	5	4	6	2
5	4	1	2	3	6
6	3	2	5	4	1
1	5	6	3	2	4
4	2	3	6	1	5

Sudoku 8

2	6	5	4	1	3
3	1	4	6	2	5
5	2	1	3	6	4
4	3	6	2	5	1
1	4	2	5	3	6
6	5	3	1	4	2

Sudoku solutions

Sudoku 9

6	1	3	4	5	2
5	4	2	1	6	3
2	3	1	5	4	6
4	5	6	2	3	1
3	2	5	6	1	4
1	6	4	3	2	5

Sudoku 10

5	1	4	2	6	3
3	6	2	5	4	1
4	2	1	3	5	6
6	5	3	4	1	2
2	4	6	1	3	5
1	3	5	6	2	4

Sudoku 11

6	1	3	4	5	2
4	5	2	1	3	6
2	3	4	5	6	1
1	6	5	2	4	3
3	4	1	6	2	5
5	2	6	3	1	4

Sudoku 12

4	5	3	1	2	6
2	1	6	5	4	3
6	2	5	4	3	1
3	4	1	2	6	5
5	3	4	6	1	2
1	6	2	3	5	4

Sudoku solutions

Sudoku 13

3	2	1	6	5	4
6	5	4	1	2	3
1	3	5	2	4	6
2	4	6	5	3	1
5	1	3	4	6	2
4	6	2	3	1	5

Sudoku 14

6	5	4	1	3	2
1	3	2	4	6	5
5	1	6	2	4	3
2	4	3	5	1	6
4	6	5	3	2	1
3	2	1	6	5	4

Sudoku 15

6	4	5	1	2	3
2	1	3	5	6	4
1	2	4	3	5	6
3	5	6	4	1	2
5	3	2	6	4	1
4	6	1	2	3	5

Find two same pictures

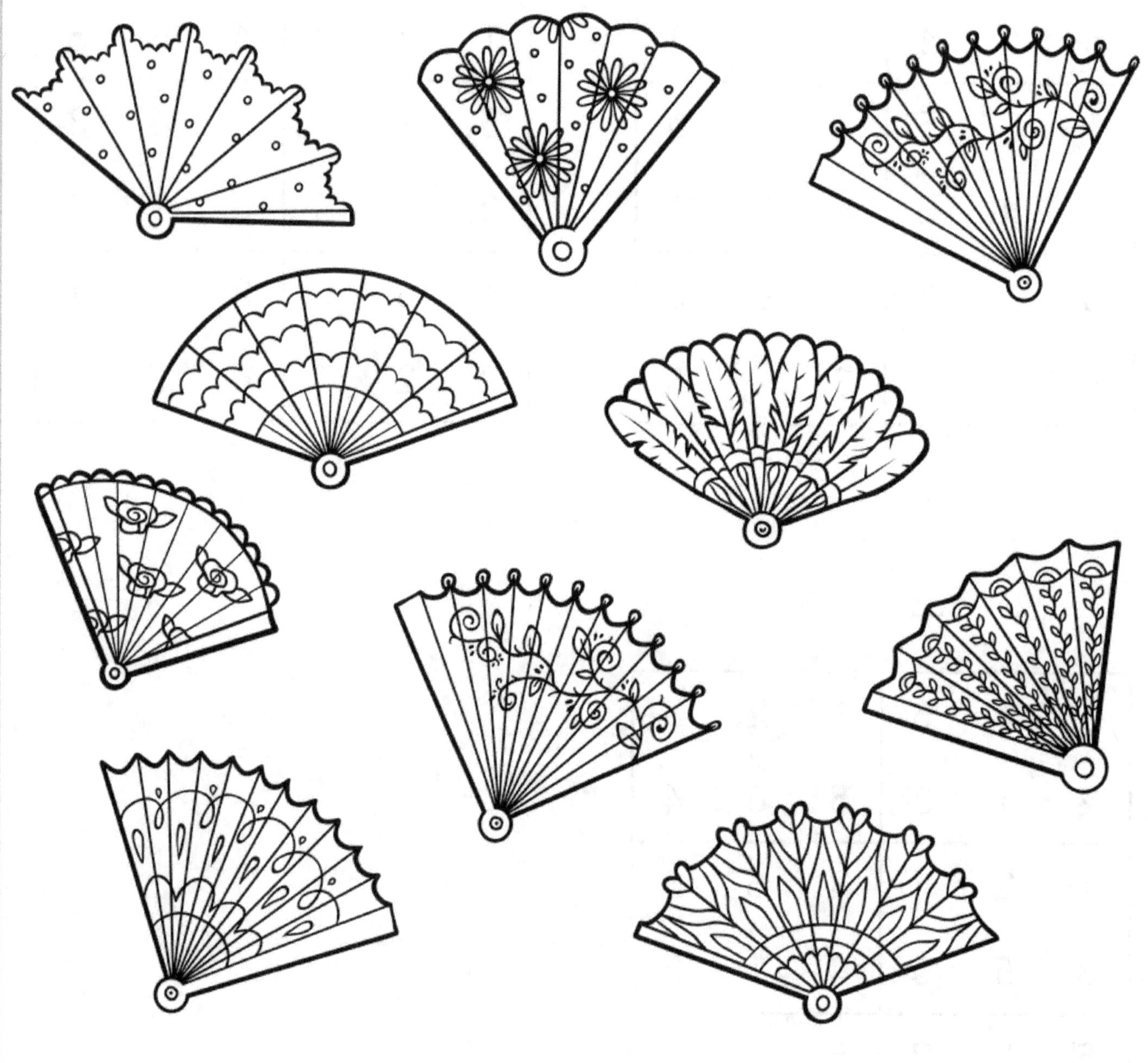

Find two same pictures

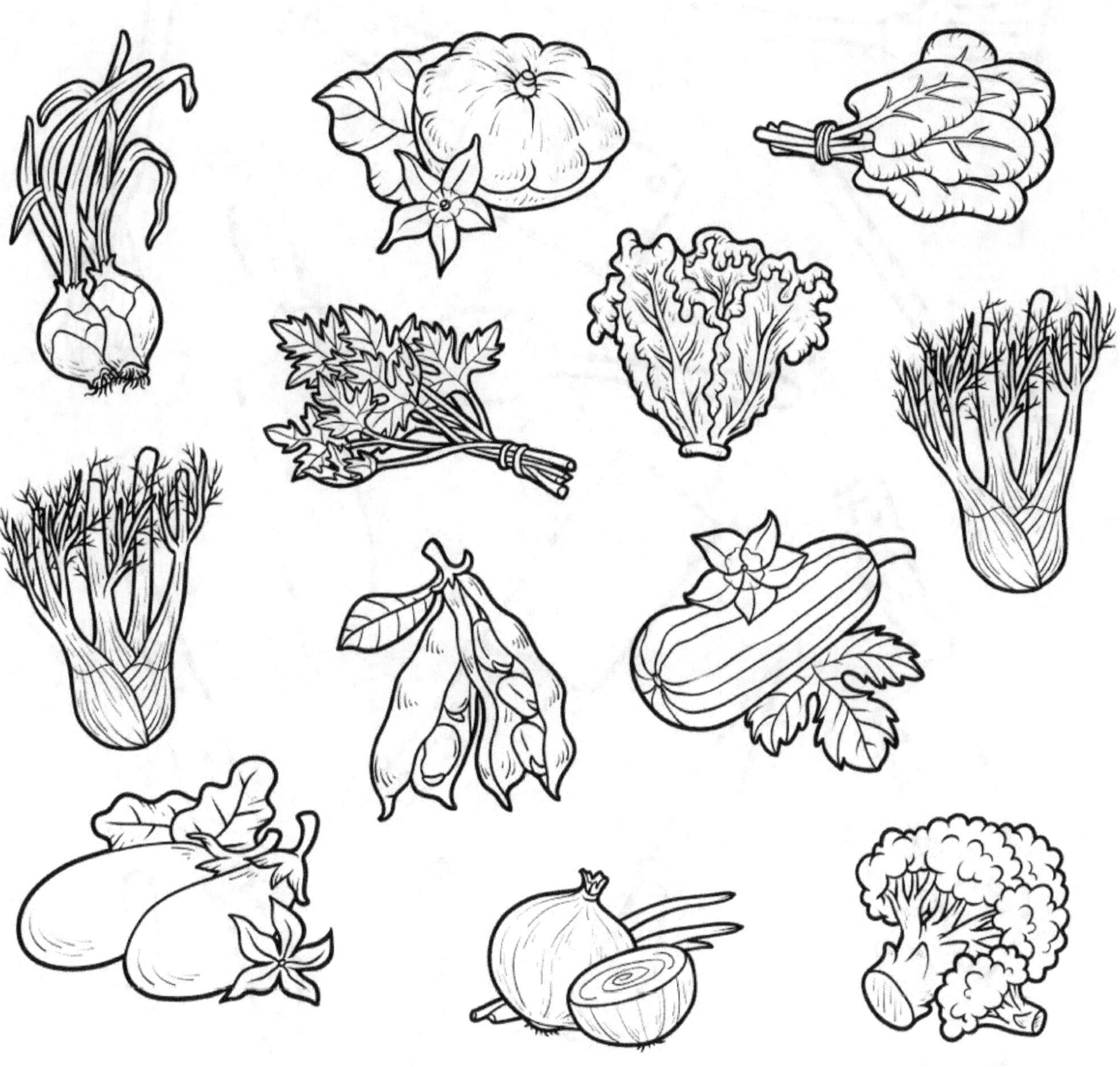

Find two same pictures

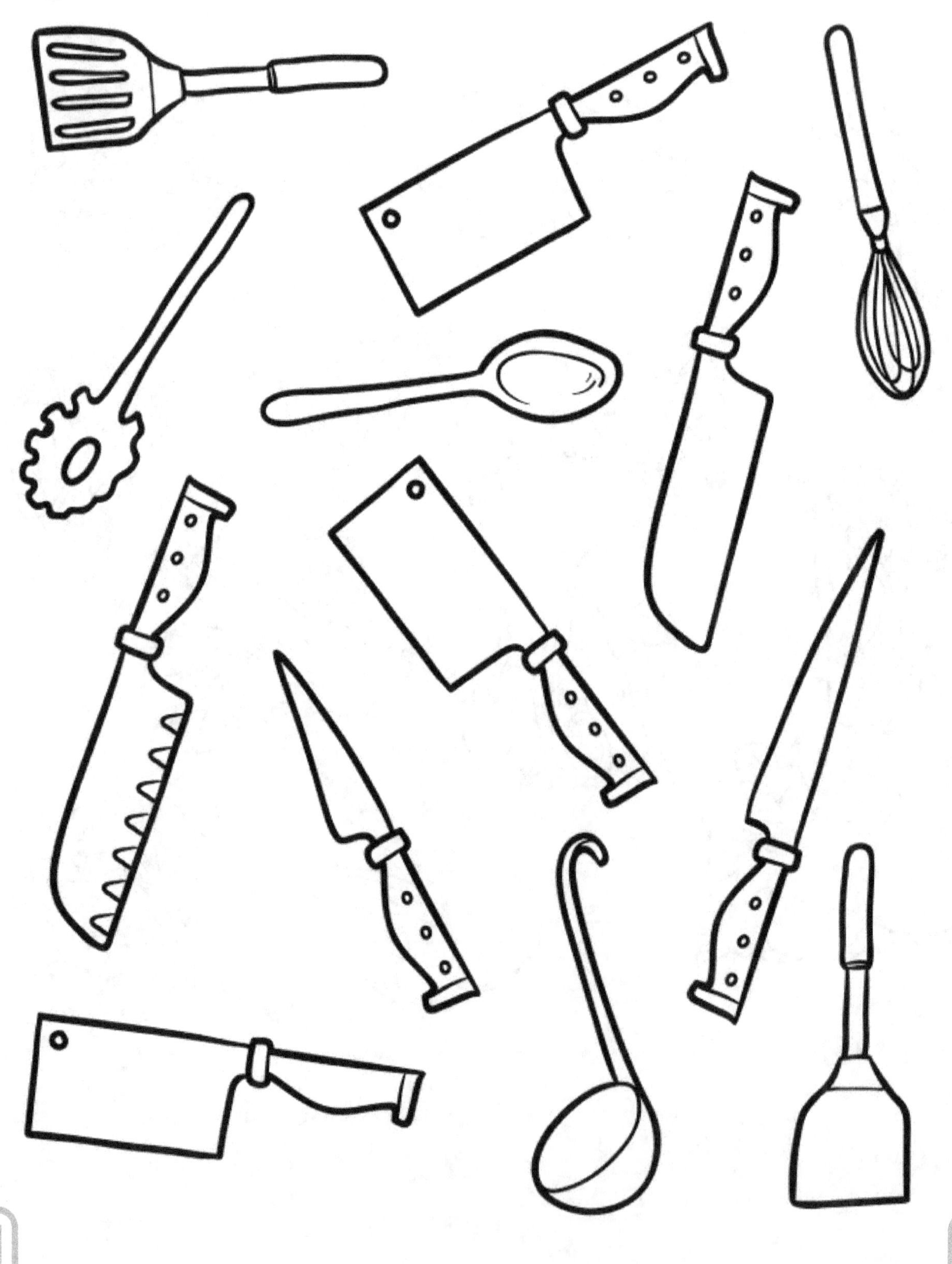

Find two same pictures

Find two same pictures

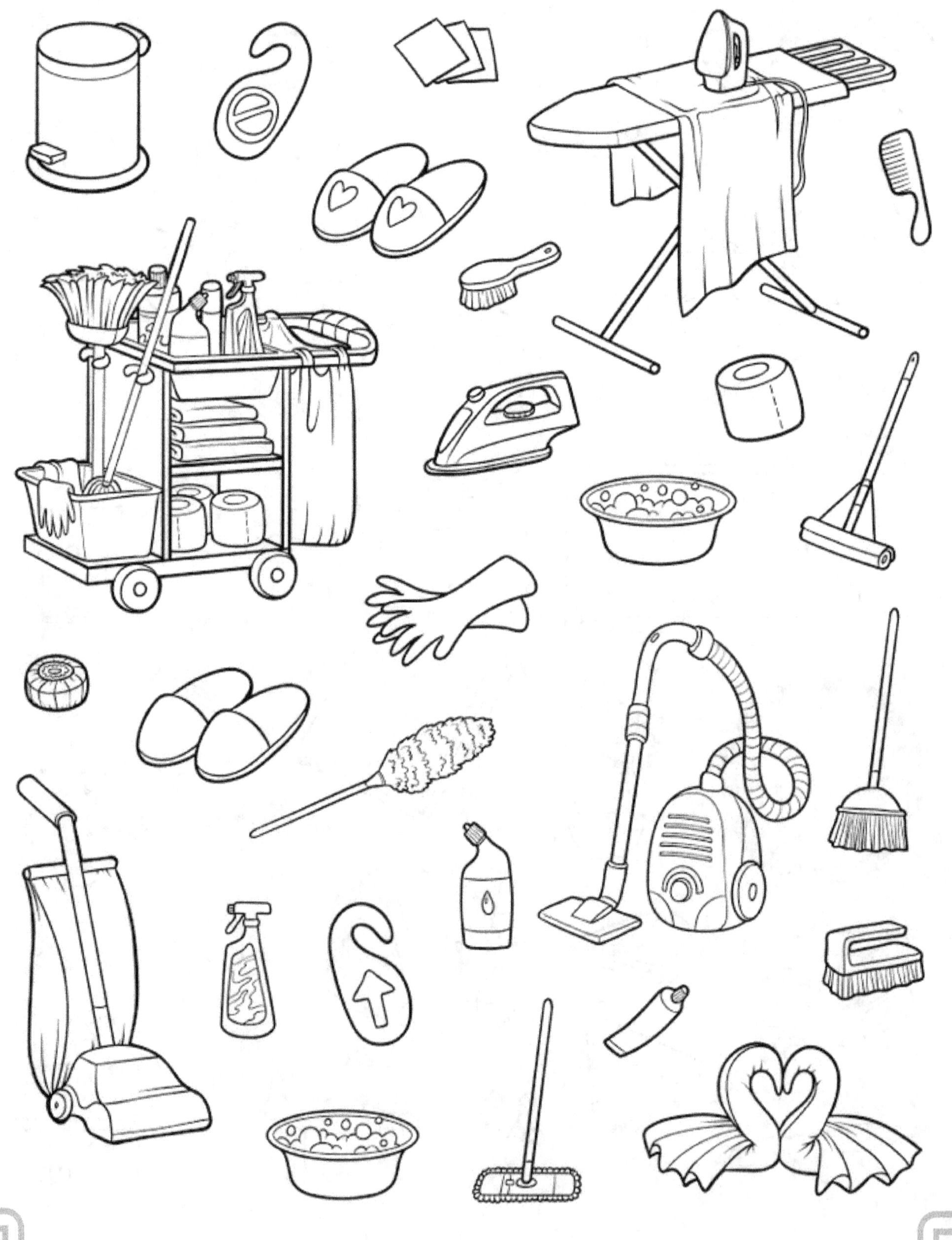

Find two same pictures

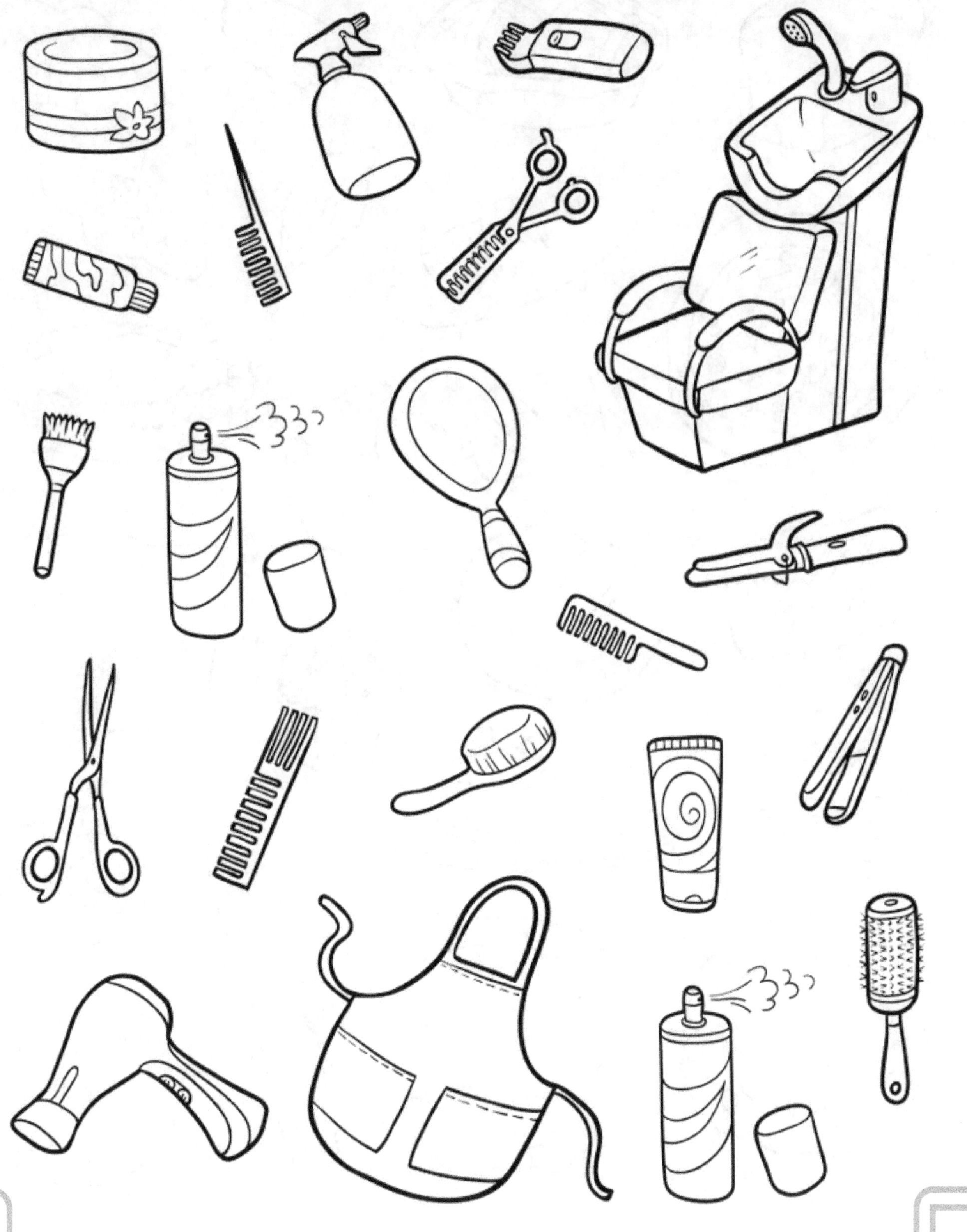

Find two same pictures

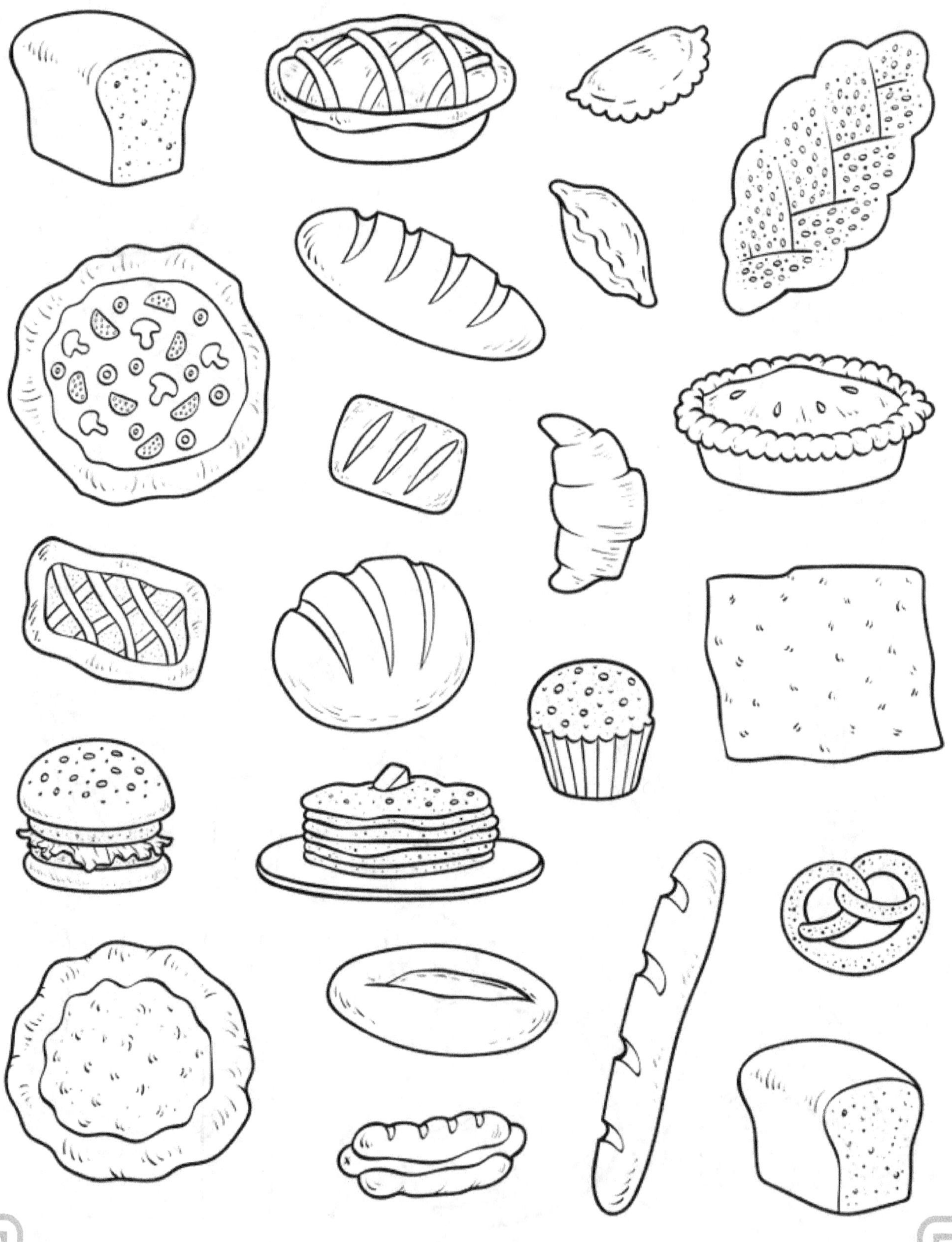

Find two same pictures

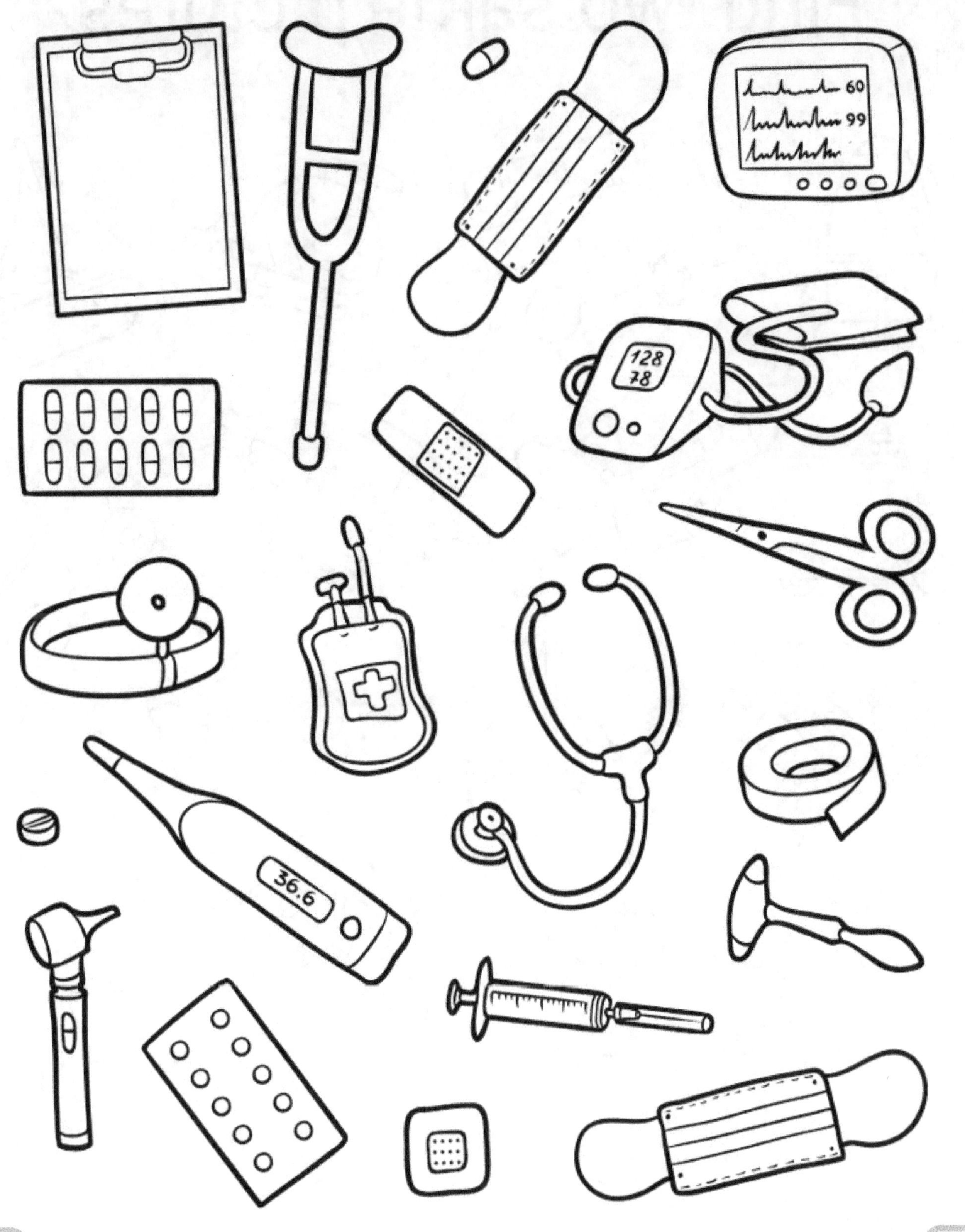

Find two same pictures

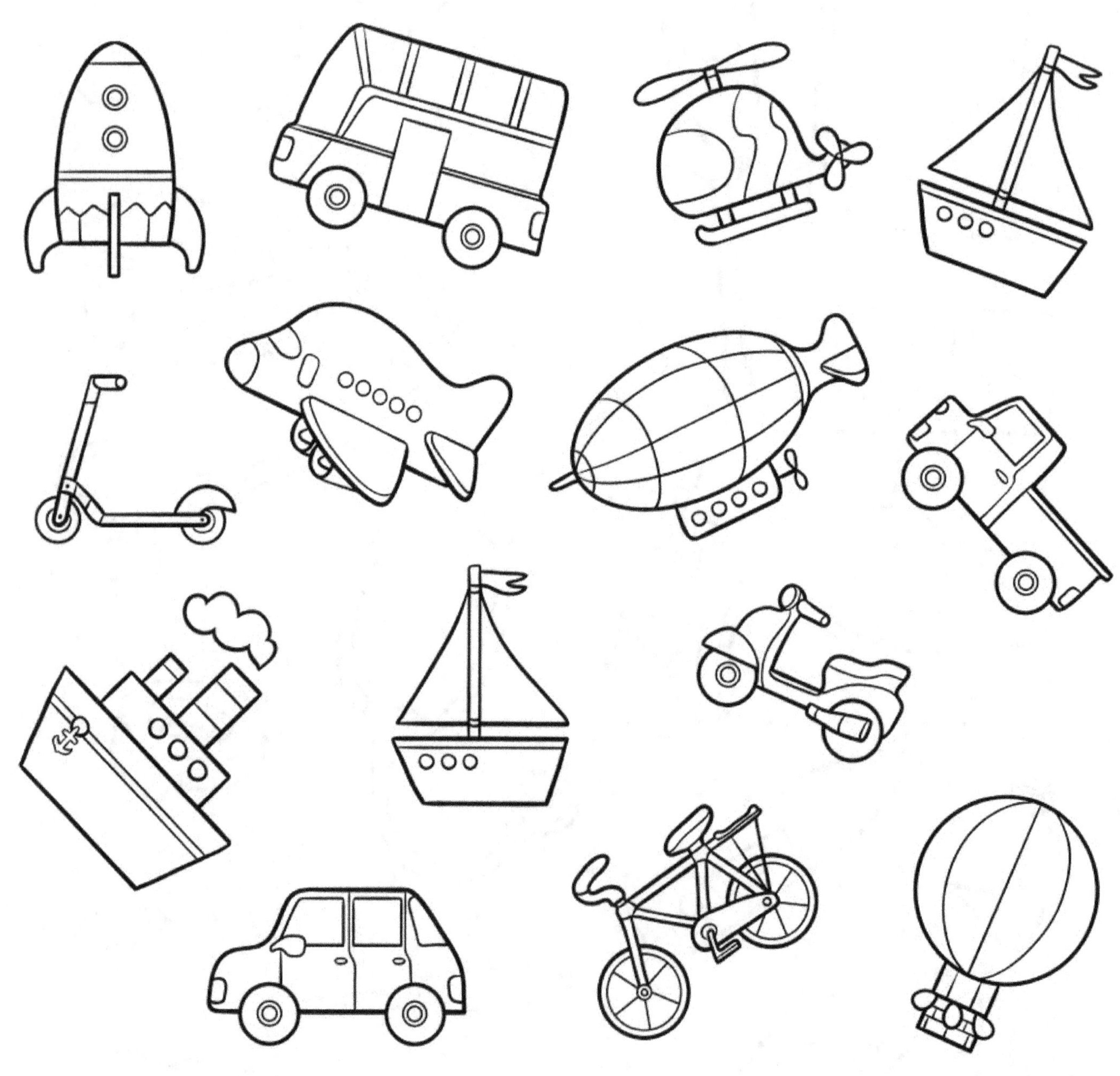